Advance Praise for Mindfire

"*Mindfire* perfectly sums up and dives into accounts of navigating your twenties—which has its highs and lows—and adds the layer of mental health. By having these discussions, we not only normalize the conversation, but foster connection and healing. The rawness and transparency makes this book an invitation to acceptance and openness."
—CHARITY LAWSON, *The Bachelorette, Dancing with the Stars*

"This book is so important to so many. We need to realize anxiety and OCD are not just words, but real, debilitating medical issues that so many people experience."
—HOWIE MANDEL, comedian and OCD advocate

"I was so impressed to hear Carrie wrote a book detailing her mental health journey. Mental health struggles can feel overwhelming and scary to talk about, so I applaud Carrie's vulnerability and fearlessness."
—LAURA MARANO, actress and star of Disney's *Austin and Ally*

"As a parent of a teenager, I applaud Carrie's bravery in sharing her mental health struggles. Our youth need to know that they're not alone and it's OK to ask for help. Thank you for being a bright light for mental wellness, Carrie."
—MEAGHAN B. MURPHY, Editor-in-Chief of *Woman's Day*,
   author of *Your Fully Charged Life*

"It's so exciting to have young people, like Carrie, starting more of these conversations surrounding mental health. She's keeping it real in a digital age where we so often forget that others are sharing similar struggles."
—KYLIE CANTRALL, actress and star of Disney's *Descendants: The Rise of Red*

"I've overcome many mental health battles myself, and Carrie's deep dive into the struggles of the mind makes me feel seen. I'm not alone—and neither are you."
—RUBY MCAULIFFE, Associate Commerce Fashion Editor at *InStyle*

"Mental health now more than ever needs advocates who have firsthand experience. Social media guru Carrie Berk knows firsthand how difficult the hurdles of mental health in a society centered around internet presence can be. Growing up in the vortex of an ever-changing frontier from COVID to political unrest and more, Berk speaks from experience and continues to be an avid advocate for all young adults."
—JULIA REMILLARD, writer for *Daily Mail*

"As we grow up, oftentimes, we forget to put ourselves first and check in with how we are feeling. Carrie does such a great job at balancing work with moments of joy. Her book helped me learn more about how to stay healthy mentally."
—KATIE FEENEY, TikTok and YouTube Star

"I believe mental health and wellness are so important for young adults. Carrie Berk is a wonderful advocate for helping young adults learn how to regulate their feelings and behaviors."

—Kristin McGee, former Peloton yoga instructor

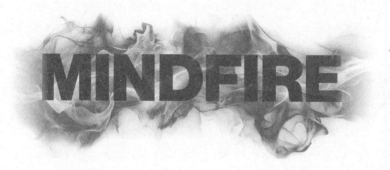

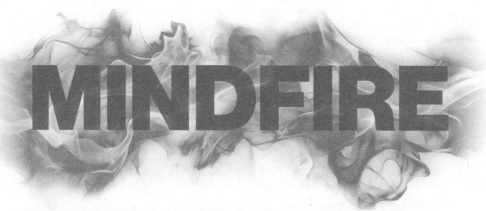

MINDFIRE

DIARY OF AN ANXIOUS TWENTYSOMETHING

CARRIE BERK

Post Hill
PRESS

A POST HILL PRESS BOOK
ISBN: 979-8-88845-958-4
ISBN (eBook): 979-8-88845-959-1

Mindfire:
Diary of an Anxious Twentysomething
© 2025 by Carrie Berk
All Rights Reserved

Cover design by Daniela Hritcu
Cover photo by Nigel Barker

This book, as well as any other Post Hill Press publications, may be purchased in bulk quantities at a special discounted rate. Contact orders@posthillpress.com for more information.

Post Hill Press
New York • Nashville
posthillpress.com

Published in the United States of America
1 2 3 4 5 6 7 8 9 10

I love you, OCD.

I love how you never go away.

I love how you occupy endless hours of my day.

I love how you're never satisfied.

*I love how you make it feel like
my brain is in overdrive.*

I love how you rise with the sun and are never done.

I love how you make me question who I am.

*I love how you make it seem like my world
has been shaken and slammed.*

I love how you make me ruminate.

*I love how you put my mind on loop so that
double-checking constantly makes me late.*

I love how you make me scared.

*I love how you make me feel unworthy
when I'm not prepared.*

*But most importantly I love how you
taught me how to be strong.*

To fight my own battles.

Although living with you, the fight's already been won.

-CARRIE BERK

TABLE OF CONTENTS

INTRODUCTION

Trigger warning: self-harm/suicide/depression

What does it mean to be happy? I used to think it meant utter and complete peace of mind. Going about your day-to-day business with no stress, no concerns, and most importantly, no anxiety. To me, happiness was a superpower. It meant being able to look at life and only focus on the positive. Anything potentially negative or hurtful would just fade into the background.

That all changed when I turned eighteen. I blew out my birthday candles, and for the first time in my life, I was scared of growing up. I looked around me: it was mid-December and snowing hard in the depths of the COVID-19 pandemic. Life seemed dull, dark, and hopeless. I was not happy, and I didn't know if I ever would be again. I forgot what it felt like to smile. The childlike spirit I harbored in 2019 was now lost. I was lost.

I experienced my first panic attack in August 2020, but I now realize my anxiety journey dates back long before that. I was eight years old when I first experienced OCD symptoms, even though at the time, I didn't know it. Everything had to be even on both sides. If I touched a table with my right hand, I had to touch it with my left hand, too. I'm not sure what brought this on, but once my brain convinced me of the need for balance, it wouldn't stop. The urge for these motions to feel "just right" was agonizing. It delayed everything—washing my hands, eating my dinner, doing my homework. I was barely functioning. My mom and I made up a name for this habit. We called it "qua qua." The name was deliberately silly so that what was going on seemed less serious. But I was lying to myself—it was debilitating.

I made it stop by setting an ultimatum. I told myself that if I didn't stop doing "qua qua," everyone I love would get hurt. It was a superstition. Not even—it was a lie. But for eight-year-old me, the prospect of hurting my family was enough to make me stop. Just like that, there was no more "qua qua."

I didn't have any OCD surges until ten years later, when I began to approach adulthood. It was the summer of 2020, in the middle of the pandemic. Life as we knew it came to a halt. What I dealt with seemed minimal compared to the global losses due to COVID-19. For me, it started off with school being paused for two weeks. Then prom got canceled, followed by graduation indefinitely postponed. There was so much uncertainty about our futures—would these milestones be rescheduled? Would we see our friends again? How were we supposed to kickstart our college careers if we were trapped inside our homes in quarantine? My math final was canceled after I studied for over a month. My internship offer was rescinded. My upcoming travel plans to L.A. were no longer possible. Everything I looked forward to was no longer a possibility. I was blindsided.

According to a KFF/CNN survey, fifty percent of young adults (ages 18-24) reported symptoms of anxiety and depression in 2023 following the pandemic. Another recent study from the American Psychology Association found that Gen Z is more likely (27 percent) than millennials (15 percent) and Gen X (13 percent) to report their mental health as fair or poor. Who wouldn't be anxious if their entire life was suddenly enveloped in disappointments and fears during such pivotal years?

My family and I retreated to our summer house on Long Island in 2020 and stayed for over a year. We had little choice—New York City was shut down. There were food, water, and toilet paper shortages, and even a curfew. I remember sitting on the couch a few months before my eighteenth birthday, eating a cup of cereal while watching an '80s rom-com with my mom. All of a sudden, my breathing became shallow. I put down my cup on the couch, nearly spilling the milk, and started gasping for air. I became hyper-focused on my breathing. My surroundings didn't feel real anymore. I looked intensely into my mom's eyes to ground myself as I told her, "I can't breathe."

My heart began to pound. I was terrified. My mom held my hand and guided me through eight-five-eight breathing: in for eight seconds, hold for five, out for eight. It didn't help. She took me upstairs and gave me my inhaler (I keep one just in case because of my cough variant asthma). I sat upright in her bed and held her hand, trembling and hyperventilating. I had no idea what was happening to me. This sensation was strange and unfamiliar.

The next day, my parents took me to get a COVID-19 test. It was only a few months into the pandemic at this time, so we didn't know much about the illness. We just assumed I caught the virus. To my surprise, my test came back negative. "Maybe it's just anxiety, honey," my mom proposed.

I always thought anxiety and stress were synonymous. Now, I know there's a notable difference. Stress is often a direct response to a situation, while anxiety can be caused by something that doesn't exist or is not currently happening. My anxiety wasn't tied to anything, but somehow, I couldn't shake it. Every night for two months, I couldn't go to bed without trouble breathing. I'd wake up every morning with a pounding heart and shaky hands. Sometimes, I'd be so jittery and unfocused, I would drop my breakfast on the floor. It became the new normal. I was sick of running to my mom confused and in tears. "What's happening to me?" I wailed.

Unfortunately, things did not get better from there. One dreary afternoon at a pumpkin patch, a friend confided in me that she had been so anxious and depressed, she started cutting her wrists. She rolled up her sleeves to show me her scars as she spoke. The world fell silent. I was numb. "Is this what happens to people with anxiety?" I wondered.

From that day forward, I couldn't shake that thought. I convinced myself that I had anxiety, and people with anxiety eventually hurt themselves. It's not true, nor did I want to hurt myself. But my OCD wouldn't let go of the thought. I had a lot of trouble functioning. I couldn't ride my Peloton without tearing up over instructors' words: "You woke up today. Fix your face" or "My Pelo-heart believes in you." I would sit at the edge of my bed, staring at the ceiling as my brain did cartwheels trying to logic its way out of the anxiety. "You don't want to kill yourself because you love life" was the recurring escape thought. I had rehearsed and memorized my answer. But the thoughts were never neutralized. My OCD was not convinced.

The anxiety turned into depression. I would rarely leave my bed. The routine: sleep, exercise, eat, repeat. I would fold in some filming for my TikTok to keep me busy and distracted. It made me feel alive. Not to mention, the constant praise and steady follower gain gave me an endorphin boost. But it was only temporary.

One day, the constant rumination became so exhausting, I collapsed over my Peloton bike in tears and called my mom over. "I can't do this anymore," I said. "I need help." My mom was worried I was suicidal, which made matters worse. I mean, it's understandable. Why would her daughter think about suicide all the time if she wasn't contemplating it? I swore to her over and over again that I wanted to live. I wanted to be happy. But the more the negative thoughts stuck, the more real they seemed, and the more both my family and I believed them.

My mom found me a therapist whom I started seeing in December 2020. I had seen a therapist briefly when I was fourteen to deal with an eating disorder, and the experience was traumatizing. Asking for help made me feel weak and powerless—why couldn't I just solve the issues by myself? That first therapist gave me an ultimatum: she wouldn't continue to see me if I didn't work with a nutritionist. I was angry, disgusted, and very hurt.

I had told this woman more about my life and my mental demons than anyone ever before, and she was treating me like a robot patient, not a human being. After her, I swore I'd never see a therapist again. I convinced myself they were solely in it for the money.

It took me reaching the lowest point I'd ever hit in my life to reach out for help. I knew I needed a therapist. Nobody could force me to get one. At first, meeting with her was difficult. Not only was I skeptical about her intentions, but she also made me face my problems head on. There was no more pushing them down or pretending they weren't there. Soon after I started seeing her, she officially diagnosed me with generalized anxiety and obsessive-compulsive disorder (OCD).

THERAPIST'S COUCH:

GENERALIZED ANXIETY DISORDER

*According to Nathan Peterson, OCD Therapist
and Licensed Clinical Social Worker*

Generalized anxiety disorder (GAD) is different from temporary stress. A person with GAD feels anxious all the time, even when there's no clear reason to be worried.

They may feel overly worried about several areas of life: health, family, job, finances, school, or relationships. The distress continues for an extended period and may feel like too much to handle. A lot of the time, someone with GAD feels anxious without even knowing why they're anxious. They worry about one thing before it suddenly switches to something else. It's a never-ending cycle.

Someone with GAD may experience physical and mental symptoms: being on edge, growing tired easily, or struggling to concentrate. Their body might ache more than usual, and they could have trouble sleeping. While anxiety is designed to warn us of real danger, the anxiety felt from GAD can make the person feel like the danger is valid, even if it's a false alarm. Many times, the fears stem from uncertainties. We don't know the future, which causes the brain to get stuck in a loop of anxiety. It moves from one feared topic to another in waiting for an answer that may never arrive. It feels like your brain is doing you a favor by warning you, but these are things you don't need to be concerned about. Ruminating over them becomes less of a help and more of a hindrance.

THERAPIST'S COUCH:

OBSESSIVE–COMPULSIVE DISORDER (OCD)

According to Kimberley Quinlan, LMFT, Anxiety and OCD Therapist

Obsessive-compulsive disorder is a chronic mental health condition characterized by persistent, recurring obsessions and repetitive compulsions performed to alleviate the anxiety, uncertainty, or discomfort caused by these obsessions. Compulsions can be physical behaviors or mental acts. OCD can significantly interfere with daily life, relationships, and overall well-being. Research shows that approximately 1-3 percent of the population has OCD. However, we are not sure how accurate these statistics are given the stigma of mental health and difficulty attaining access to health care and correct diagnosis.

OCD affects people of all ages, races, and sexual orientations, with symptoms often emerging in childhood or adolescence. The exact cause remains unknown, but genetic, neurological, behavioral, cognitive, and environmental factors are believed to contribute to its development. Stressful life events and changes can exacerbate symptoms. Living with OCD can be challenging, but with proper treatment and support, many individuals can manage their symptoms and lead fulfilling lives.

My therapist led me through exposure therapy to desensitize me to my intrusive thoughts. It was very difficult. I told her that because of my intrusive thoughts, I was sensitive to certain objects tied to self-harm, like razors, knives, and pill bottles. One exposure we did was staring at a photo of a razor for five minutes. Afterward, she would ask me what my SUDS were ("Subjective Unit of Distress Scale"). I had to rank how distressed I was feeling on a scale of one to ten before, during, and after the exposure. One of the more difficult exposures was placing a razor on my wrist and staring at it for an extended period of time. A level up from that was placing the razor on my wrist, staring at it, and actively thinking about the intrusive thought at the same time. I left each session feeling highly distressed. My therapist would recommend doing something to keep me busy afterward (exercise, film TikToks) or calm me down (smell lavender essential oil). I kept telling myself, "Short term pain, long term gain."

For a while, I was scared of sharing my intrusive thoughts aloud with my parents because I didn't want them to think they were true. If they got upset, it would validate the OCD and make my thoughts seem like something to worry about. For a later exposure, my parents joined a therapy session as I read a couple of intrusive thoughts aloud to them from a sheet of paper. I was instructed to look them in the eye as I said the words, "I want to kill myself." It hurt me deeply to say something I didn't believe but was on my mind. I could see how much it hurt my parents, too. Their eyes anxiously darted around the room as they struggled to stay composed.

Although exposure therapy was hard, I looked forward to each session. Talking to my therapist validated my feelings. She never punished me for my thoughts. It felt like she was the only person who really understood. We met virtually twice a week for forty-five minutes. I would count the days between appointments. Living in between the sessions was lonely. I became reliant on my therapist to make me feel safe in my own skin when I didn't feel capable of doing that myself. The thoughts running through my head made me afraid. I didn't know who I was anymore.

Most days, I'd wake up in tears because the same intrusive thought was still there. I was beyond frustrated. Anxiety stripped all the color from my life. I couldn't have fun without feeling the thoughts in the back of my head. When I looked in the mirror, I didn't recognize myself.

The world around me was a blur. I would force myself to feel the five senses by naming objects around me or smelling strong aromas. It helped ground me to the present. I tried my best to go about my normal life, but the reality was, I felt anything but normal. I look back at photos now—smiling, playing in the snow, running around the Met Museum with my best friend—and see behind my eyes how much I was hurting.

I struggled for about six months before I really hit a turning point. I can't remember the exact moment, but I remember coming to the conclusion that my anxiety was not going to go away. I wasn't trying to be pessimistic. I was finally being pragmatic. I needed to stop waiting for the day when I would wake up and no longer feel anxious. If you check for your anxiety, it will be there. Once I started expecting the anxiety and intrusive thoughts, I wasn't as scared of them. They became "normal" because I was used to them. I panicked less when thoughts persisted. I was so overexposed to them, I became desensitized. I put so much work into exposure therapy that one day, the intrusive thoughts just vanished. I realized that no matter what was burdening me, I still made it through the day. I learned by living.

So, where does that leave me now? It's been over three years since that anxious episode at age eighteen (what I like to call the start of my adulting era). My anxiety is by no means gone. Over the past few years, I have dealt with new intrusive thoughts and different challenges with my anxiety. As my life has shifted, so have the thoughts. The content varies. Family, relationships, religion, violence, and germs/contamination are all common OCD themes. I've also cycled through different compulsions: checking and rechecking if an email was sent, deleting photo out-takes from my camera roll, and even triple-checking for typos in this very paragraph. I've cried, but I've also conquered a lot.

Writing has always been a form of therapy for me. When I'm trying to make sense of what's going on in my mind, I write down everything I'm feeling. My therapist's number one recommendation when I'm in the middle of an anxious episode is to start journaling. I like to think of it as "writing my way out" (to quote *Hamilton*). However, my mission for this book is more than just a means of self-therapy. I hope to increase society's understanding about anxiety and OCD because the disorders can be painfully misunderstood. Some people joke about being "so OCD" when there are people genuinely impaired by it. They treat OCD like a quirky personality trait when in reality, it can be very intense. They don't know how destructive their ignorance can be.

I can do my part in spreading awareness and sharing my story, but the issue is institutional. There is not enough mental health education in schools. I took a "Natural Science" class my junior year of college, and we spent one day discussing mental health. OCD was brushed over after a mere minute of lecturing. The examples given for OCD were excessive cleaning and organization. A stock photo of someone scrubbing a table was shown on the smart board. It was just so wrong—so incomplete. OCD was misrepresented, as was I. We need to do better.

I'm not saying there hasn't been any progress. OCD and anxiety used to be taboo when my parents were younger. Fifty years ago, people thought going to therapy meant there was something wrong with you. Case in point: when my mom was having panic attacks in high school, seeing a psychiatrist was a threat rather than a helpful suggestion. My grandma told my mom it was where all the "crazy kids" go.

Today, it seems like everyone has a therapist. Therapy is talked about more in mainstream media, as is anxiety. But apart from people saying how important mental health is to them, I haven't seen many personal stories shared publicly, particularly from the perspective of young adults.

So what do I want? What's my objective? I want to feel understood, as I'm sure many others with anxiety and OCD do as well. I want people to educate themselves and try to understand what it feels like to function while your mind is on fire. To go to work while your anxiety is already working overtime. To set goals when mental illness tries to stop you.

It all goes back to increased education, and not just through what you see in medical journals. The more we talk about mental health, the less shame there is attached to it. People sharing their genuine experiences can change the narrative of what OCD looks like in the media. No, it's not Khlo-C-D (Khloe Kardashian's self-proclaimed obsession with cleaning her house and color-coding her pantry). Speaking up is challenging. I'm doing my part by being vulnerable in this book. But I can't carry the weight of the world on my shoulders. This is your story. This is our story. We're in this together—the future is in our hands.

I wanted to publish this series of diary entries I've written over the past few years so that those of you who are currently struggling can see you're not alone. Each chapter is defined by a powerful word or emotion I've experienced in hopes that you feel heard and empowered. A person with OCD craves reassurance; I'm not going to tell you why your thoughts aren't true. Instead, I hope you see yourself through my words and realize relatability is far more powerful than reassurance. I hope you recognize that anxiety does get better. It did for me, and it can for you, too. Every day will not be perfect, but growth is possible.

You know that feeling the second you drop from the peak of a roller coaster? It's intimidating, exhilarating, and absolutely terrifying all at the same time. That complexity of emotions is the best way to describe how I'm feeling right now as I sit in my bed to write this (I've never been much of a desk girl). It feels incredibly rewarding to know that being open about my struggles might move people. But I'll be honest: putting my darkest moments on display for everyone to see is scary.

I want to clarify that I am not a therapist or psychologist, nor am I an OCD expert. I'm just a normal twenty-two-year-old who suffers from generalized anxiety and OCD every day. I'm an expert on my own life and I can speak with vulnerability and truth about my personal experiences. In a sea of doctors who study mental health, sometimes all you need is a normal girl candidly telling you how she feels. Sit back, get comfy, and let's get real.

Note: With the exception of the example provided in the introduction, I chose to omit the contents of my intrusive thoughts in this book, and that is intentional. Telling readers the specifics of each intrusive thought is a form of confession. That would be letting the OCD win. It's never about the specifics of each individual thought—it's about the anxiety surrounding the disorder.

CHAPTER 1

TRAPPED

As I sit here ruminating, I'm stuck in a memory. The scenes run through my head in an endless loop. Sights and sounds of the past become tangible. The present fades into the background as I'm taken back in time, transported into my former self. I'm not very good at remembering things, even from the year prior. The memories that are closest are those that hold the most emotional significance.

Let's rewind to 2010. I'm eight years old, laying on my bed, and it's been hours since I curled up in the sheets to sleep. The culprit: OCD. My self-proclaimed "qua qua" held me captive. Every time I started to fall asleep, I remembered that I only touched my nightstand with my right hand, not my left. Or I cracked my back on one side and forgot to do the other. Everything needed to be even on both sides. I wasted so much time and energy on nonsense. I was only eight. I had so much life to live. OCD was draining it from me.

Research shows that it takes fourteen to seventeen years on average for someone to receive an OCD diagnosis. When I see that data, I see eight-year-old me, and I'm sad. I wish I could go back and hold her hand. Why didn't anyone help her? Why did it take so long to get answers? I thought I was going insane because my symptoms were foreign to me. That's not fair to a little girl who was just trying to be a kid. I should have learned about my anxiety and OCD much sooner—through school, a therapist, or my parents.

I think about the feelings chart that was hidden in the guidance counselor's office at my elementary school. It taught kids about different types of emotions they might be feeling: sad, excited, scared, confused. Mental health education can start with something as simple as that: teaching children how to identify their emotions and accept them for what they are.

The guidance counselor's office was reserved for special needs kids. It wasn't necessarily welcome to all students. I never really got to look at that feelings chart other than a quick glance when occasionally delivering the guidance counselor's mail. The concept of talking through my feelings with an adult seemed taboo at the time when it should have been encouraged. You were sent to the guidance counselor's office if you got into an argument in the school yard, or if you sounded off to the teacher in the classroom. There was a preconceived notion that this was where the "bad kids" went. It became a principal's office of sorts when really, it should have been a safe space for kids to visit when they wanted to discuss their feelings. I wonder if my school had provided greater education on mental health, if I would have been diagnosed and learned how to cope with my OCD much sooner.

We should normalize listening to kids who express that they need help. I'm not saying to force them into therapy prematurely. Start by simply providing a listening ear. Gently guide them and explain under-the-surface emotions from early on—what does anxiety look like? What does it feel like? It's not just kids who need to be educated. It's parents and teachers as well. Adults must join the learning curve to prevent misinformation from being spread to children. That may look like mandatory health training for educators in the future. We need to make sure people, especially kids, are not improperly diagnosed.

Recently, I ran into a past school counselor at the hair salon. I never actually went to visit her after class, but I recognized her face. I spun my chair around to face her and introduced myself as a former student. We caught up on what I had been up to, and then I asked how things were going at school. "We're living in a mental health crisis right now. You have a huge responsibility to help students," I said. Her face turned pale. She was speechless. "Yeah…" was all she managed to utter before she quickly shuffled out of the salon. It was as if she felt like she was guilty. She knew she wasn't doing enough to help students with their mental health. It was a shame, really. I could see by the blank look in her eyes that she knew what she needed to do, and she was embarrassed it wasn't already being done.

Our parents and grandparents grew up in a world where anxiety and OCD weren't really discussed. It's up to us to take the reins over how mental health is handled in society. Without people speaking out, mental health will continue to be taboo. Eight-year-old girls will continue to suffer in silence like I did. I was too afraid to ask for help. I had to fight my way through OCD all by myself. I knew how much it was stifling me, so I eventually managed to move past my symptoms. My eight-year-old self was much smarter than I give her credit for. Nobody knew how much she was struggling, yet she persevered. Even though she was young, she pulled herself out without any help. She's a superhero.

I'll be honest: I do still engage in a rotation of physical compulsions. I'll listen to songs repeatedly so I can reflect on their lyrics and fully understand what they mean.

I'll hoard information from magazines and newspapers, reading advertisements and articles from cover to cover. None of this is necessary, but OCD dictates otherwise.

THERAPIST'S COUCH:

OBSESSIONS VS. COMPULSIONS

*According to Kimberley Quinlan,
LMFT, Anxiety and OCD Therapist*

Obsessions are repetitive, unwanted, and distressing thoughts, images, emotions, sensations, or urges. Obsessions can target any area of one's life. They range from fears of contamination, symmetry, concerns about safety, morals, religion, and relationships to intrusive violent or sexual thoughts. Despite recognizing these thoughts as irrational, individuals with OCD often feel powerless to stop them, leading to significant uncertainty, anxiety, and distress.

Compulsions are physical behaviors or mental acts performed in response to the obsessions. These actions aim to reduce one's experience of discomfort or prevent or reduce the likelihood of one's feared event. Compulsions are commonly excessive, take up a significant degree of time, and impact one's functioning. Common compulsions include physical acts such as washing hands, checking locks, or counting or moving objects. Compulsions may also involve avoidance, mental compulsions, self-punishment, and reassurance seeking. The relief provided by compulsions is typically temporary, creating a cycle that perpetuates the disorder.

Arguably, there's nothing more compulsive than skin picking. When I'm engaged in mental or physical rumination, I pick my knuckles until they bleed. I'll tell people it's from a boxing session or that I have eczema. It's particularly embarrassing when someone is hesitant to hold my hand, or when a stranger offers me a Band-Aid on the bus. I'm not intentionally trying to harm myself. It's a mindless act, a means of self-soothing, if you will. No matter how nasty my skin looks (or how much hand cream I apply), I have a hard time stopping.

Another draining physical compulsion stems from the anxiety journal I keep in the Notes app on my phone. I'm always writing things down to talk about in my therapy sessions, no matter where I am or what I'm doing. Yesterday, I was walking my dog and stopped to write while she was peeing. I forgot to retract the leash, and she nearly got run over. I'll think of things to write at the most inopportune times. When I'm on my Peloton, I keep my phone across the room for that very reason.

The bike is my safe space. I'm locked in with no distractions. When I'm clipped in, my mind and body are free. I walk away with more insight about living a positive, fulfilling life than the thirty minutes before I pressed play. My Peloton saved my sanity during the pandemic. When life was at a standstill, it gave me something to look forward to every day. It provided a break from my intrusive thoughts and inspired me to pick up the pieces of my life. It has also played a key role in helping me cope with OCD compulsions. During the hour I'm sprinting in the saddle or performing intervals on high resistance, there's no time to obsess.

That said, I often find myself rushing to the Notes app right after my ride, spilling out several paragraphs. Even when I finish writing, I'll read my work over and over again. In my mind, the notes must be perfect. They need to be organized, make sense, and have perfect grammar. I'm not sure why it matters; nobody sees these notes but me, not even my therapist. Because of my OCD, my mind isn't at peace until the sentences before me are "just right."

Sometimes, I'll even interrupt my shower. The other day, I stood naked in my room, conditioner dripping from my hair and onto the floor, as I typed on my phone. The shower was still running. The hallway that connected the bathroom to my bedroom was soaking wet. But I told myself that if I didn't write my thoughts down right then and there, I wouldn't remember them. That feeling made me uneasy.

Although the things I write are conversation topics for therapy, a lot (okay, most of it) is random, irrelevant, and unnecessary. I feel the need to write down every musing that crosses my mind: why am I craving more hugs from my dad lately? Why did my best friend call me less this week? Why does my face look rounder than it did a year ago? My OCD convinces me that everything needs an answer. I ruminate over each and every question that's raised with paragraphs in my Notes app. Still, I never reach a resolution. With compulsions, you never do. It seems like you're working toward a solution to your thoughts, but in reality, you're just wasting time. Every question that strikes doesn't need to have an answer. It doesn't need to be written down, nor does it need to be overanalyzed. Thoughts are meant to flow freely. You don't need to stop and reflect on each one. You can be mindful that the thought is there and allow it to exist without judgment or resistance.

I find comfort in the fact that compulsions come and go. The compulsions I once performed when I was eight I no longer even consider. Looking back at the physical compulsions now has actually helped me better come to terms with my anxiety and OCD. When I start questioning intrusive thoughts and wonder if they're real, I remember how OCD is a part of who I am, and it has been for a long time. The physical compulsions led me to better understand the mental compulsions and accept them for what they are: a disorder.

Instead of panicking, I try to be patient with myself. Finding hope in the small wins has been a huge help in getting physical compulsions under control. I recognize that progress can be subtle. It's not always visible, but that doesn't mean it's not there. I celebrate the moments when I resist compulsions, like when I put my Notes app away for a certain amount of time. And when I fail, I pick myself up and try again. Some days are easier than others.

Writing on my phone is highly compulsive. I'm well aware. I'll tell friends I need a moment on FaceTime calls or stand in the middle of a shopping mall to perform compulsions. It slows me down and makes me late for appointments. It ruins my plans and precious moments with friends and family. It cuts into my sleep schedule. Performing compulsions is debilitating. I want to be present when people talk to me, but instead, my brain is in overdrive. I worry I come off as rude when disengaging in conversation. Little do my friends know, it's not their fault.

Anxiety can be overwhelming, not just to you but to those you let into your inner circle. When I first told my best friend about my OCD and anxiety, she did not understand as well as I would've liked her to. I recounted everything I'd gone through from the beginning while she sat in silence. We've been friends since I was a tween, but she was not familiar with this part of me. She saw me as a successful young woman who goes after what she wants and is unbothered by anything or anyone. Although I appreciated her support, sometimes I wished she better grasped that there's more to me than my success. You can be smiling and still struggling. You can be outgoing and still feel alone. Nobody's perfect.

As I explained to her what intrusive thoughts are and why they burden me, she didn't blink. She listened politely and carefully. I could tell she was taking in all the information as best as she could, but it was new to her. No matter how many times I told her that intrusive thoughts are contrary to your personal beliefs and desires, it didn't seem to resonate.

THERAPIST'S COUCH:

INTRUSIVE THOUGHTS

According to Kimberley Quinlan,
LMFT, Anxiety and OCD Therapist

Intrusive thoughts are unwanted involuntary thoughts and images that can be disturbing and distressing. These repetitive thoughts often pop into one's mind without warning, causing significant anxiety and discomfort. While everyone experiences occasional intrusive thoughts, for someone with OCD, these thoughts can grow persistent and seem more important than they actually are.

Intrusive thoughts can take many forms, including violent, sexual, blasphemous, or harmful themes. For instance, a person might have an unwanted thought about harming a loved one, even though they have no desire to do so. These thoughts do not reflect the individual's true feelings or intentions, but can lead to intense fear and self-doubt.

The nature of intrusive thoughts can vary widely among individuals. Common types include:

- Harm-related thoughts: Worries about accidentally causing harm to oneself or others.
- Sexual thoughts: Unwanted and distressing sexual images or urges.
- Religious or blasphemous thoughts: Fear of committing a sin or offending one's religious beliefs.
- Contamination thoughts: Excessive fears about germs or dirt leading to compulsive cleaning behaviors.
- Relationship thoughts: Uncertainty and doubt about the fidelity or love of a partner or the fear of not truly loving one's partner.
- Symmetry or "just right" obsessions: Discomfort and distress when objects are not arranged in a specific order, "in their right place" or symmetrically, or when things feel "not just right."
- Health-related thoughts: Uncertainty or fear of having a serious illness.

The key challenge with intrusive thoughts is their persistence and the distress they cause. For those with OCD, these thoughts often trigger compulsive behaviors or mental acts aimed at neutralizing anxiety, uncertainty, and distress.

> Unfortunately, these compulsions typically only provide temporary relief, reinforcing the cycle of intrusive thoughts and compulsions.

She asked me why my anxiety was any different from stress. I think of stress as more of a short-term struggle with explicit triggers. For example, panicking over turning in a work assignment on time, or getting jitters before a presentation. I know exactly what my anxiety feels like and how it manifests through intrusive thoughts. So when stress strikes, I immediately sense the distinction. I often like the stress more because it makes the anxiety seem quieter. I feel like I have more control over my stress, since it's centered around real concerns that I can address and take action over. Anxiety tends to be more intense and continual. It also doesn't necessarily have a trigger. Eating, sleeping, and breathing as a young adult is enough of an explanation for having anxiety.

Although anxiety and stress might manifest similarly (fatigue, lack of focus, rapid heart rate, insomnia), they are notably different. Many people aren't aware of the difference. That's part of the reason anxiety is so misunderstood, especially when it lingers. I can't tell you how many times people have asked me "why are you still anxious?" as I go about my day. Some will say, "why don't you just think a different thought if it bothers you so much?" It's not so simple to set your brain back on course. Thoughts are generally out of our control. The idea is to accept the thought—no matter what it is—instead of suppress it.

When I told my other best friend about my anxiety, she understood completely—almost to a fault. When I sat her down in 2020 to talk about it, she was also struggling. "I'm so scared. When is this ever going to stop?" I cried. She shook her head and squeezed my hand. "I don't know. I've been in therapy for eight years," she said. I was terrified. I was going to feel like this for eight years? How was I supposed to survive?

I loved that I had someone to talk to about my anxiety. The problem was that it became everything we talked about. Whenever we hung out, I knew I was in for a crying session. We would sit on the couch all day, watch TV, and mope. I started to forget the last time we laughed together. Instead of boosting each other's spirits, we pulled each other down into a deeper pit.

Learning how to talk about my anxiety productively with friends has been a struggle for me. Everyone reacts differently, so it's difficult to prepare for the conversation. It's gotten easier as time has passed and I've become more comfortable with my mental health. In 2020, when I was still learning about anxiety and OCD, talking to people who didn't get it made me feel worse. It made me feel damaged or "diseased." Now that I have a better understanding, it's easier to explain my anxiety to others. You don't have anything to prove to anyone. The friends that don't care or make an effort to be there for you are not worth holding onto anyway.

I've slowly shown my friends my anxiety—whether intentionally or accidentally. One day, I was having an anxious morning, but I had picnic plans with a few friends on someone's patio in the afternoon. I pulled myself together to go—food and friends would surely boost my spirits. But as everyone gave life updates, I was completely depersonalized. I saw mouths moving, but their words were not registering. It was as if I wasn't even there. My brain was entirely elsewhere. Everyone was having fun while I was in my head and miserable.

THERAPIST'S COUCH:

DEPERSONALIZATION

According to Dr. Robi Ludwig,
NYC Psychotherapist

Depersonalization is a common symptom of anxiety. Those who feel depersonalized are disconnected from their thoughts, feelings, and sensations. Depersonalization can make you feel like you're watching yourself from outside your body. It can make it seem like things around you aren't real, as if you're in a fog or lost in a dream.

This feeling typically occurs when your brain is stressed. It's a defense mechanism that the brain uses to protect you from dealing with too much emotion. When a person is feeling really anxious or stressed, their brain might disconnect from their thoughts and feelings to cope with the overwhelming emotions.

I stayed quiet, stuffed my face with chips and guac, and let my friends lead the conversation. I tried to focus on what they were saying to bring myself back to reality, but my brain had other plans. The more they spoke, the more my anxiety brewed behind the scenes. Eventually, I couldn't hold it in anymore. I told everyone I had to take a phone call and stepped away from the table. I hid behind a tree and once I was out of sight, I broke down into a full-blown panic attack. I couldn't think straight, nor could I gain control over my breathing. I was all alone and helpless. I wished I could walk back to the table, tell my friends what was going on and ask for help, but I wasn't comfortable doing so. I was close with them, but not to the point where I wanted to expose this side of me.

Eventually, I texted the one friend I trusted at the picnic to bring me my bag so I could go home. It was the only option. I didn't want to return in tears and suddenly become the center of attention. Besides, the girls were not aware of my anxiety, and I wasn't in the right headspace to explain it to them right then. My friend brought the bag, and she sat next to me for a few minutes as I cried onto her shoulder. She asked why I was having a panic attack, and I didn't know how to answer her. There was no explicit trigger in this instance. I'm not sure she understood, but she provided a safe space for me to cry.

Although I've started talking about my anxiety publicly, I still get scared bringing it up to my friends. The conversation is more personal. These are the people I care most about, whose opinions I value wholeheartedly. The best way I go about talking to them about anxiety is to lead with an educational edge. I wait until a time when I'm not too emotional to explain in detail. Going into depth when I'm already vulnerable leaves me at risk of feeling even worse if they don't accept my anxiety. I love leaning on friends when I need a shoulder to cry on, but saving the lengthy explanations for later is ideal.

I'm also aware that they may ask a lot of questions. They may not understand anything you're talking about.

The key is that they try to understand so they can be a better, more supportive friend. They do their research and make you feel like your voice is heard. You shouldn't feel criticized for opening up. If you feel the slightest bit judged, you can take the liberty of respectfully leaving the conversation. Stepping away for the sake of your mental health doesn't make you a coward. If anything, it makes you strong.

If you want to talk to your friends about OCD, there is such a thing as saying *too* much. Revealing the content of your intrusive thoughts can be counterproductive. It can scratch an itch when OCD is telling you the thoughts are important and need to be shared. In reality, these are thoughts you don't need to attend to. Instead, you can focus on describing how you're feeling and what emotions you're cycling through when your brain is loud. Choosing to disengage from an OCD thought is not a weakness; it's a smart, conscious choice. It's not avoidance; it's deliberate disconnection to better your mental health. There's a difference between pushing thoughts down and accepting them, then letting them fly over your head. The goal is the latter.

You know who you are better than anyone else. Befriend yourself first. Your friends should be there for you when you need them, but at the end of the day, you should be there for you. Work on understanding yourself then share as much as you feel comfortable with others. And remember, you're not crazy. You're just human.

SELF-CARE CORNER:

ASSEMBLE YOUR TRIBE

Something I learned in middle-school science class still resonates: Einstein said that energy cannot be created or destroyed, but it can be transferred from one form to another. I often refer back to science as context for my anxiety. When anxiety dims my light, I recall that the energy to move forward was inside me all along. It was never destroyed—it just needs to be harnessed.

But sometimes, channeling that energy from within is easier said than done. That's when your tribe comes in—family, friends, and loved ones who provide some of their energy if they see you're struggling. Asking for help doesn't make you weak. Having a team of people behind you to call upon when you're at your worst supercharges you. It's a sign of strength to admit that you can't do it all yourself. Surround yourself with positive people who lift you up, and filter out those who do the opposite.

I've lost friends over my anxiety because they didn't make any effort to understand what I was going through. They believed self-care is selfish. The reality is that not everyone is going to get it. But there are people out there who will see you for who you are and be there no matter how you're feeling in the moment. Build a tribe of people who make you feel comfortable being unapologetically yourself. Let them hold you up until you can stand on your own. Then march forward.

CHAPTER 2
PANIC

I just ran the TCS New York City Marathon, and it was everything and nothing like I expected. I trained for eight months to conquer the grueling hills and bridges that come with the feat. But the greatest challenge wasn't the Queensboro Bridge as anticipated. It was a panic attack I suffered at mile twenty-one.

For the first twenty miles, I was flying. I kept a steady pace and was confident my training leading up to the November race had served me well. Temperatures reached a record-high of seventy-five degrees with high humidity, so I stayed hydrated. I didn't think the heat would affect me. But as I climbed up the Manhattan Bridge, I got nauseous, and it hit me: what if I don't finish this marathon?

A fear of failure triggered a full-on panic attack. It felt like I couldn't get enough air in my lungs. I stopped in the middle of the bridge, folded over, and hyperventilated. Runners rushed by me, and it felt like I was standing in the eye of a hurricane. I was all alone with my thoughts. My phone wouldn't work because it was soaked with sweat, so I couldn't even call my family for support. I was the only person who could bring myself to finish that marathon.

I ran the previous nineteen miles with a friend, but I didn't want to hold her back. "I'm having trouble breathing. Go ahead of me, it's okay," I insisted. She grabbed my hand and made me promise I would finish no matter what. I promised, but truthfully, I didn't know if I could get there. All the miles behind me seemed like nothing compared to the final ten kilometers. I had run 10K hundreds of times before. It's crazy how one panic attack can jeopardize everything you've worked for in just a moment.

While I was running, I recalled the first time my mom told me she experienced a panic attack. She was in a toy store and suddenly got dizzy. She sat on the ground while someone brought her a pack of M&Ms to elevate her blood sugar. The cause of her panic: unknown. Panic often comes unannounced, and you're left wondering what you did to deserve the sudden burst of anxiety. I felt similarly during the marathon. Sure, I was attempting an unbelievable feat. But I was doing fine: my legs felt great, my stomach didn't hurt, and I was eating and drinking plenty. My anxiety seems to creep in during the moments of my life that matter most: a career high, a beautiful vacation, a birthday. It only made sense that it arose during the marathon. When things are going according to plan, it's as if an alarm goes off in my head that alerts anxiety to emerge. It's unfair, but it's life.

Less than a mile after I started panicking during the marathon, I saw my aunt's brother waiting for me on the sidelines as I crossed back into Manhattan. He held a hot pink sign that said "Carrie On." I felt pressure to smile as I approached him, but I couldn't control my emotions. I started crying hysterically. "I can't breathe. I can't breathe," I repeated. He told me to inhale through my nose and out through my mouth, but the surrounding cowbells and confetti cannons made it difficult to focus. "Stop and walk a bit until you find your footing," he said. I shook my head. My running coach was right up ahead. I told myself I needed to pull it together.

So I kept running with tears streaming down my face. Onlookers cheered me on as I ran down Fifth Avenue. I couldn't soak in the crowds or appreciate how exciting it was to hear them screaming my name. The intrusive thoughts telling me I might fail were so loud, I couldn't focus on anything else.

I was humiliated by my uncontrollable crying. I broke down in front of family, friends, and even strangers managing the water stations at every mile. Everyone told me my emotions were nothing to be ashamed of, but I didn't listen. I envisioned myself smiling the entire race and soaring over the finish line, and I was upset that wasn't my reality.

So, I finished the marathon. I didn't get the final time I expected. I didn't enjoy the last six miles. Plus, I vomited twice and fainted after I crossed the finish line. But I've realized that this race meant much more than that. I signed up because I wanted to prove to myself how strong I am—not just physically, but mentally.

I recalled why I started running in the first place. It was the beginning of the pandemic, and I felt lost. My typical modes of exercise—SoulCycle, Orange Theory, Rumble Boxing—all shut down. Life was paused. I didn't know what was going to happen next. Running was my constant. When my brain was screaming with intrusive thoughts, I forced myself onto the road and just started running. The sun was shining, and the path ahead seemed endless. I blasted an outdoor running class on my phone and persisted. I pretended I was running toward peace of mind. For the hours (yes, hours) I was running, my head was clearer. I was invincible. Even though my anxiety would return when I got home, for a while, I was free. To this day, when my anxiety is brewing, running centers me.

A surprise panic attack during the marathon was the ultimate test of mental strength. I could've stopped completely, sat on the side of the road, and hailed a taxi. But I kept going. I walked for a few intervals to catch my bearings, but I ran across that finish line. I was determined to not give up.

Funny enough, I think I might run another marathon. Those 26.2 miles felt like an impossible battle to overcome. It was me versus me out there. The loud cheers from the crowds raised my spirits, but they didn't carry me forward. That was all me—mind, body, and spirit. The marathon served as a poignant lesson that helped me view my life in a new light: at the end of the day, you will always have you. When life gets difficult, you have the power to look within yourself, dig deep, and rise above. You can reach out to others for a helping hand, but the strength to change your situation, the ability to grow and flourish, all starts with you.

When I was experiencing that panic attack, I felt stuck. My legs were hardly aching, but my brain was screaming to stop. The mental game was far more difficult than any physical challenge I endured throughout the course of the race. Yet the beauty of the marathon is that you just keep going. When things get hard, your body goes on autopilot, and you keep putting one foot in front of the other. My mind may have been a mess, but my body was doing what it was trained to do. I was proud of the work I put into preparing to take on the race.

The marathon was an out-of-body experience. I was depersonalized from my surroundings for the last few miles because I was so adamant about finishing. I hate that my most vivid memories from the race were when I was suffering. However, I look back at videos people took of me from mile twenty on, and even though there were tears in my eyes, I was still running. I may have been slower than when I started, but I was still moving. I proved to myself that I can get through hard things. I'm stronger than my anxiety—and I have the gold medal to prove it.

Author's Note: When this book went to press, I had just run my second marathon. I felt strong, triumphant, and incredibly proud. Not to mention, I didn't have a panic attack.

SELF-CARE CORNER:

FIND YOUR FITNESS

Before I found running, I was a dancer for fourteen years. The environment was extremely toxic: bratty ballerinas, teachers poking at my feet on pointe, and pressure to stay skinny to conform to the dancer stereotype. I hated it, but it was all I knew. I was afraid to quit because I didn't know who I was without dance.

I'm forever grateful that I found running. The pandemic lockdown forced me to get outside and try something new. I am so glad I did, because now, I have no idea who I would be without it. Running makes all the anxiety, stress, and chaos of the outside world fade away. Everything, if only for an hour, feels like it's okay. Nothing and nobody can touch me. When I'm pounding the pavement in a park or along a beach boardwalk, I feel the most like myself. Running gives me a passion and purpose when it feels like all other hope is lost.

Fitness is a powerful tool if you choose to harness it. Moving your body is medicine. Find what movement works for you. Due to the outside pressures I faced, dance was clearly not a good fit for me, but running feels like home. Whether you choose to practice lower-intensity exercise (yoga or pilates) or cardio (running or cycling), getting your heart pumping is a certified way to boost endorphins. It allows you to channel your anxiety productively and teaches your brain that you will not and cannot be stopped. Intrusive thoughts may leave my mind feeling paralyzed sometimes, but I refuse to keep my body stuck. On days when it's hard, I force myself to pedal on my bike. I run a robotic four miles at a slower pace. I take a long walk home instead of riding the subway. Even though my brain might be screaming, I know I'll feel better after I exercise. I move through the pain because I know the sense of pride on the other side will be worth it. I know it can be tough to get motivated, especially when anxiety chains you to the couch. Try your best to think about both the physical and mental reward you'll receive after completing a workout. Exercise adds years to your life and life to your years.

Start small: move your body for ten minutes every day. It can be as simple as a full-body stretch or a walk to the grocery store. Over time, you might notice yourself start to crave movement more. Treat fitness as an adventure. There are endless classes and types of workouts to explore. If you keep an open mind, you might just discover a new passion—and boost your mental health in the process.

CHAPTER 3
MEMORIES

I hate Christmas. Call me Scrooge, but I can't help the way I feel. I've hated the holidays for the past two years because during the 2020 holiday season, I was in a depression. Anxiety and intrusive thoughts burdened me every day. I couldn't pick my head up off a pillow to face my OCD-ridden reality. I've come a long way since then (time, therapy, and an overall dedication to finding happiness). Distance from 2020 has allowed me to reflect on that experience and analyze it as if I'm talking about someone else. The further it fades into my past, the more separate it feels from my story.

Memories can be painful. Emotions rush through you, as if you're experiencing them for the first time. Whenever I remember something specific to my anxiety, something dark, it hurts. I can't think about how far I've come when the pain of the past possesses me.

When I woke up today, I remembered something that upset me. The sudden recollection was unexpected and alarming. I wasn't ready to interact with those memories. But they kept coming—one after the other, no matter where I was or what I was doing. I had forgotten some moments even happened, and this was my first time thinking back on them.

THERAPIST'S COUCH:

ANXIETY VS. DEPRESSION

According to Nathan Peterson, OCD Therapist and Licensed Clinical Social Worker

Studies show that around 60 percent of people with anxiety will also experience depression, and vice versa. Although anxiety and depression can coexist, they are fundamentally separate struggles. Depression can make you feel sad, hopeless, and tired. You might lose interest in things you used to enjoy, have trouble sleeping or eating, and find it hard to concentrate. To be diagnosed with depression, these feelings must last most of the day, nearly every day, for at least two weeks. They must also cause significant distress or impairment. Genetics, life experiences, and low serotonin levels may be associated with depression.

Anxiety is more centered around fear. You might feel nervous, on edge, sweaty, and shaky with ruminating thoughts. Anxiety doesn't like to live in uncertainty. This is why the brain may constantly warn of potential danger to keep us safe. It often produces false signals, attempting to problem-solve something that doesn't have an answer in the present moment. Constant "what if" questions leave someone stuck in the cycle of anxiety.

Treatments for both anxiety and depression may consist of challenging unhelpful thinking styles, exposure and response prevention, mindfulness, and behavioral therapy. A combination of time and treatment will ensure that each condition is regulated properly so that the individual sees improvement.

It's Christmas Day. I'm being bombarded with Christmas posts and messages. I live in New York City, home of the iconic Rockefeller Center tree and ice skating rink. Carolers are roaming the streets. The Christmas overload is overwhelming. It all takes me back in time to 2020, and I start to remember. I remember how I built a snowman outside and baked cookies to distract myself (I don't even eat cookies). I remember watching the snow fall outside my window as I hid inside, merely going through the motions. I remember hopping on the Peloton to numb the pain, although I felt just as bad when the endorphin high came down afterward. Even though I rode for over an hour, the anxiety returned as soon as I clipped out. Today, as I did the same, I fell back into a sad, quiet, trance-like state. I see the holidays as the backdrop for when I was at my worst. But it's been two years. My brain hasn't been like this for a very long time. Why today? Why again?

As I sat inside a restaurant for Christmas brunch with my family, "Silver Bells" played on the radio. My heart started to pound uncontrollably. The string of Christmas lights on the walls was blinding. I grasped my mom's hand while the host led us to the table. Music holds memories. I closed my eyes and fell down a rabbit hole, away from reality. Unlike Alice in Wonderland, I landed in my memories.

Songs bring up old emotions. Memories of years past suddenly feel like yesterday. Sorrow and fear wash over me. Music is a time machine. It has the power to elicit feelings that you didn't know you had, or perhaps you forgot. It helps you process emotions for better or for worse.

The feeling of déjà vu during an anxious episode is underrated. Today, my brain naturally wandered back to when I was at my lowest. I woke up in the morning, stared out the window, and hoped that today would be different—then felt my heart begin to pound and the cycle start all over again. I forced myself to breathe, to meditate, to find the strength to get out of bed—barely making it to the bathroom sink without feeling my heart in my throat. I couldn't seem to shake the overarching feeling that everything is wrong in the world. Everything around me seems so big while I feel so small. As I moved through the bones of my morning routine, my body felt light, as if I were moving through my life as a ghost of myself.

I can't begin to describe how frustrated, embarrassed, and ashamed this makes me. After so much progress, I'm scared that today, I feel the same as that eighteen-year-old girl did: trembling, terrified, and ever-so-anxious for no apparent reason. It feels like I've taken one step forward and three steps back. I'm sick of telling my loved ones like a broken record that I'm anxious. I want to talk about the things that make me excited in the world: marathon running, the fact that I'm approaching senior year of college, my upcoming book release, and so much more. But excitement and gratitude are stunted by anxiety. I can't seem to pull myself out.

I feel like I'm rushing to feel better—yes, because I'm eager, but also because I don't want my loved ones to get tired of hearing about my anxiety. I worry they'll become emotionally exhausted from constantly lifting me up and supporting me when I'm low. Rest assured, I would do the same for them. But I feel guilty for falling back into this pattern when I've come so far.

The anxiety cycle is generally the same for me. It starts with physical panic symptoms—short breaths, sweaty palms, a rapid heartbeat. Then, it shifts to an intrusive thought. None of it makes sense—it never does. I know I'm not supposed to try to comprehend it, but when I try to leave the anxiety alone, it still feels like there's a rock sitting inside my head. That's the thing about OCD: thoughts that weigh you down are not as easy to let go of as the average person. It doesn't mean I don't want to. Just one week ago, I was the happiest I'd been in a very long time. It's as if in saying that aloud, I jinxed myself. Why is it that the second we start to feel happy, something turns for the worse?

I'm aware that Christmas was my trigger, but that isn't always the case. Oftentimes, I don't have an answer as to what triggered my anxiety, nor does anyone else. I can be rational and talk about the anxiety symptoms I have, but as for what sparked the physical and mental compulsions, I'm at a loss. The intrusive thought doesn't cause the anxiety. It's just an anxiety symptom.

My therapist tells me to sit with the anxiety, to accept intrusive thoughts for what they are and move forward.

But doing so is uncomfortable. Intrusive thoughts are like a rollercoaster you just want to end. It seems impossible to focus and function. I don't feel sorry for myself. It's frustrating. It's not 2020 anymore. The world is back to semi-normal, so shouldn't I be normal? There are so many wonderful things going on in my life—I just ran a marathon, and my solo debut book is going to be announced soon. This is the most inconvenient time for my anxiety to creep up on me. I'm not sure whether to scream or cry.

I want to pinpoint the holidays for kickstarting my anxiety, but I feel like I'm the one to blame. Going into December, I anticipated feeling anxious. I "looked" for my anxiety. "I hate the holidays," I'd repeat to friends and family, grunting at every Christmas tree and rolling my eyes when holiday music started playing. Christmas Day is quiet; all the stores are closed, the streets are empty, and the air is frozen. At the same time, my distractions—plus the activities that give me a sense of control—are missing. My friends are busy with their families, it's too cold outside to run, and my book manuscript is with the editor. My OCD spikes during the holidays because without school or work, my brain has more time to wander. Boredom feels like a curse. I had nothing to focus on today but myself. The second I internalized, I began to remember. And I panicked.

As I'm sitting here, writing on my phone in another desperate attempt to cope, I'm scared. I don't want things to revert to the way they were in 2020. Memories are powerful. You don't need to look at pictures to remember. I wish I could seize my negative memories and hurl them into the cold winter air, leaving space for new, positive experiences to take their place. That's not possible. Those sad, scary memories are always going to be there. It's difficult not to let them wash over me when they're so vivid and specific. I feel shaky and restless, just as my eighteen-year-old self did when she stared at the ceiling all day, afraid of herself and her thoughts. I hear those very intrusive thoughts begin to creep in now, reminding me that they're always there, never too far removed. They're quieter now, yet when I'm caught up in a memory, the anxiety is deafening.

No place brings me back to 2020 more than the house I stayed in (or as I like to say, rotted in) during the pandemic. It was the place where I suffered the most with my OCD. My most tangible memories of anxious episodes are tied to that place. I avoided going back for a while because I was afraid that if I did, the anxiety would return in full force. The anxious brain tends to associate certain people, places, or things as "good" or "bad." Once I labeled my house as "cursed," I had a hard time erasing that association. Being scared that something bad is going to happen doesn't make it any more likely to happen. However, I convinced myself that I would be triggered if I went back there. I didn't want to take that risk.

I understand that illogical associations are a part of my anxiety disorder. Just because I was in a negative mindset at my house doesn't mean the house itself is negative. But memories weigh heavily on an OCD brain. Facts don't always make the anxiety easier to deal with. People with anxiety have a harder time detaching from associations. I knew visiting my quarantine house would be an exposure, and that it would take time before I could handle it. Only recently—about a year after leaving the house to return to NYC—was I ready.

The trip was harder than I expected. Memories came rushing back as soon as my dad pulled into the driveway. I looked at the tall tree across from our doorstep and remembered the numerous times I escaped outdoors to cry. Every room, every object had a negative memory attached to it. The lavender essential oil I inhaled to calm down after exposure therapy was still on my nightstand. The shampoo I used after a very emotional long run sat on the shower shelf. The bed I buried myself in after a breakup—and wrote most of my book in—wasn't made. It was lived in. I remembered that I lived in it, even when it felt like there was barely any life to live. I thought I'd forgotten everything and put it behind me, but the sight of simple objects catapulted me back in time. This place is filled with pain and heartbreak. It's hard not to make that association when I visit. The memories were so much to handle. There was no way the house would ever be the same.

THERAPIST'S COUCH:

EXPOSURE AND RESPONSE PREVENTION (ERP)

According to Kimberley Quinlan, LMFT, Anxiety and OCD Therapist

Exposure and Response Prevention gradually exposes individuals to their feared thoughts or situations while preventing the accompanying compulsive behaviors they typically use to alleviate their anxiety. By confronting their fears without resorting to compulsive behaviors, individuals learn that they can tolerate the uncertainty or distress that accompanies their obsessions. The anxiety will decrease on its own. Repeated exposures help to weaken the association between obsessive thoughts and compulsive responses, ultimately leading to a reduction in OCD symptoms.

Exposure therapy is commonly done gradually and strategically. It involves creating an inventory of one's obsessions (intrusive thoughts, feelings, sensations, urges, or images) and ranking them from least to most anxiety-provoking. The individual gradually exposes themselves to these situations, often starting with those that elicit the least anxiety and moving to the most challenging exposures over time. During the exposure, the individual is encouraged to practice using distress tolerance skills and refrain from performing their usual compulsive behaviors or rituals.

I ran into my mom's bedroom and cried. "I can't handle this. I want to go home!" I said. She held me in her arms. I felt numb and weightless. My mind raced with memories, yet at my core, I was empty. We were only staying for three days, she told me, a long weekend. My dad loves our Long Island house. He skipped up the stairs to fold new shirts in his closet and laid on his bed as soon as he unpacked. I wished I were that carefree.

I stayed at the house that weekend for my dad. I knew it was important to him to have his daughter there, and I wasn't going to let myself be defeated by my triggers. My time there was far from perfect. I remained relatively quiet and stoic. I did a lot of writing. I went on beach runs. I saged the house with my mom while reciting my Haftorah portion (it was the first prayer that came to mind) to get rid of any bad juju. I was definitely anxious, but the difference this time was that I knew I was doing something difficult and did it anyway. I was proud of myself.

I aim to rewrite my relationship with the house so that triggers are eventually more manageable. I won't run away from places I associate with pain, and as a result, I will become desensitized over time. I'm aware it will be challenging. I acknowledge that tears are inevitable. I will need to be patient with myself. But I'm keeping an open mind.

Sometimes, you are confronted with thoughts or memories you can't control. Particularly when they surface for the first time in a long time, they can seem daunting and dangerous. However, a recollection of a memory doesn't necessarily mean anything. Your body could just be processing and maturing. The more you move through the tough memories, the easier they'll be to conquer the next time you remember. Although the recollections may be painful, they're just memories. They can no longer hurt you. Bring them on.

Bad memories can coexist with beautiful ones. Instead of pushing the negative associations away, I allow them to wash over me. I feel everything. I accept them for what they are and take the opportunity to appreciate the progress I've made. Progress over perfection. I may not be the same girl I was years ago, but I will always remember her. It's okay to remember. Just because your brain revisits the past doesn't mean it has to reside there.

SELF-CARE CORNER:

PUT IT IN PERSPECTIVE

It's easy to catastrophize and get lost in the worst case scenario. Racing thoughts can feel unavoidable. When your heart is pounding and your brain is loud, try to put things in perspective. It's difficult when you're submerged in panic, but pulling yourself out to examine your situation is a powerful tactic.

Stepping outside of yourself to look at your anxiety helps you see things more clearly. Once the emotions pass, make a deliberate choice to take deep breaths and disengage from the intrusive thoughts. Recognize your behavior and set a proper coping strategy to move forward. Take a bath. Read a book. Start a workout. Choose productivity over panic.

As you're putting things in perspective, consider that anxiety often has less to do with you and more to do with anatomy. Let me spell it out for you: is it that time of the month? Studies have shown that the premenstrual phase is associated with higher levels of anxiety. A spike in hormones may affect neurotransmitters in your brain such as serotonin and dopamine that regulate your mood. Certain vitamin deficiencies, autoimmune disorders, and medical conditions can also contribute to anxiety.

Not every day is going to be great. It's not supposed to be. But when you find perspective, you may realize that the anxiety isn't actually as scary as it felt when you were in the thick of it. Remind yourself of all the times you pushed past your anxious thoughts. And remember, you're not the only one struggling, even though it may feel that way sometimes.

CHAPTER 4

HEARTBREAK

I promised myself I'd never write about romance again after finishing my solo debut book, *My Real-Life Rom-Com*. I poured all my emotions onto the page. I became closer to achieving self-love and helped others in the process. The book was closed—literally. But I'd be remiss not to reflect on the profound impact heartbreak has had on me as someone who suffers from anxiety. I wanted to avoid putting this on paper again, yet I feel it's essential to include. Heartbreak is personal and painful, but it's part of adulting.

Anxiety and heartbreak go hand in hand—panic and pain become one and the same. There are so many thoughts and emotions brewing, yet all you feel is numb, paralyzed in fear over where you will turn next. Who are you without the person who made you feel whole? How do you build yourself back up when you feel so empty?

Thanks to anxiety, your heart beats faster—it won't stop pounding. Your breath gets shorter. Your hands start shaking. Intrusive thoughts and questions about your purpose and self-worth swarm your brain. It's all so loud.

Then suddenly, without warning, your heart slows down. It almost feels like it comes to a stop, as if envisioning life without that person has literally sucked the life out of you. The world has less color. Your surroundings become blurry and black and white. Your body feels weightless, like you're there but not really there. You're existing, but not really alive. And everything is silent— eerily silent.

You want to have faith. You want to believe your heart will repair. But how? When the heartbreak cuts so deep, you can't just put a Band-Aid over the wound. It's all-consuming. It can feel like the world is ending, and you don't know what to say, what to do, how to act, who to talk to. Personally, my mental health began to suffer.

Heartbreak is one of the things I fear most in this world. I've had my heart broken a few times, and I've lost myself in the process. There is a tremendous weight of worthlessness placed on your shoulders when the person you love says goodbye. Yes, it's a partnership. Yes, there are two people involved. But it can feel like you're losing a part of yourself. It's not selfish to cry. We don't cry on purpose. Crying is real. It's human. Sometimes, the tears come and they won't stop—no matter what anyone says or does. Heartbreak puts you in an extremely vulnerable state. When I got my heart broken, I felt fragile, like the mere touch of someone's hand could make me fall apart.

Speaking of vulnerability…let's talk about *sex*. I did not lose my virginity to someone I loved. Yet somehow, I left the experience feeling more heartbroken than I could have ever imagined. I understand that exploring your sexuality is an important part of adulting—no matter how scary or anxiety-inducing that may be. At twenty years old, it's only natural to loosen the reins a bit. And that's exactly what I did.

Going into my potential first time, I had never felt so conflicted. I was pursuing a friend, not a stranger. I knew it was a safe option. But was I really ready? Was he the right person to choose to experience my first time with? The moment was symbolic in my mind. It always had been.

I tried to convince myself it was no big deal. "I'm comfortable with him," I told my best friend over FaceTime. "So what if we're not in love? I'd rather lose my virginity to a friend I've known forever than some stranger." The boy and I had known each other for eight years and hooked up for the first time six months prior. Now that we were spending the weekend together in a shared hotel room, it seemed like the perfect opportunity to further explore our chemistry.

The day leading up to it, my friends had conflicting opinions about the matter. My best friend knew I would be upset afterward. The boy lived across the country. She saw how I reacted once he returned home after our previous hookup. It felt like the rug was ripped out from under me. One minute, we were in each other's arms, and the next, he was ghosting me. He tended to only text when we were making plans to see each other in person.

Some older friends told me to have fun and live in the moment. They all had sex several times before, and there was an unspoken pressure to catch up. I had just turned twenty, and it felt like I was late to the game. I was at the hair salon that morning and started tearing up as multiple friends blew up my phone with advice. The contradictory texts were overwhelming. I had no idea what to do. I didn't know what my heart wanted. The anticipatory anxiety was overwhelming. But I knew it wasn't worth getting worked up over something that hadn't happened yet. I couldn't live my life always worrying about how future me was going to feel. I ultimately decided to take the leap and deal with the consequences if they were ever to come.

So I had sex. It wasn't as monumental as I anticipated. With all the buildup, I expected the heavens to open and to see the light. It wasn't that deep. That said, he made me feel extremely comfortable. I thanked him for being such a safe space for my first time. "Of course. You deserve it," he said earnestly. At that moment, I knew I made the right choice.

As we lay there, he told me he wanted to travel the world together—Hawaii, Mexico, and beyond. He revealed that he wished he lived on the east coast so he could date me. "I wish things were different," he said. But we both knew long distance would be impossible for us. We would have to stay what I called "flirty friends" for now and see each other when we were in the same city. He woke me up to kiss me goodbye on his last day, and we ended our weekend on the perfect note.

Once he flew home, I assumed we would continue to text and FaceTime. This experience brought us closer. There was no way it would be the same as six months prior when he stopped messaging me completely. For a few days, he texted me. We spoke about how wonderful our weekend was, as well as his upcoming trip to New York in two weeks. But after some time, he started to pull back. He would leave my Snapchats on open and texts on read. There were no more flirtatious messages. His words were cold and bland.

I found out he was flying back to New York through his Snapchat story—he didn't mention when he was coming. "Thanks for telling me," I sarcastically messaged him. His response stung: "I'll let you know if I have time to see you." It seemed like I was an afterthought to him. Had our weekend together meant nothing? I pushed my emotions down to prove to myself—and to the friends who expressed concern from the beginning—that I was okay.

He was the exact same person he was when we first hooked up. Some people never change. We weren't dating, so in his eyes, there was no need to keep in touch. I wasn't expecting a romantic commitment from him, but it seemed like he wasn't even willing to be friends anymore. I had opened up to him emotionally and physically. And for what? To get my heart broken? People always leave. Not only was he gone, but he had taken my virginity, and I would never get it or him back.

It's complicated to consider whether I regret the sex. He made me feel safe when we were in the moment and intimate—that's what matters, right? I tell myself that whenever I feel tears starting to form today. I can't begin to express how much it hurts to have someone take your virginity and leave. My first time may have been comfortable, but the aftermath placed a dark cloud over that memory. I can't think about the joy I felt in the moment without considering the pain that followed. And I know for a fact he doesn't feel the same. Clearly, he's an "in the moment" type of guy—out of sight, out of mind. While the sex was a monumental occasion for me, it was nothing to him. I was nothing to him.

No matter how much I tell myself that first-time sex is no big deal, deep down, I disagree. I got caught up in the heat of the moment and surrendered to the sexual tension. It felt like it was the right time to lose my virginity. But is there ever really a "right time?" There is no right or wrong when it comes to sex, only decisions and the way you handle what happens after. When I climbed into my childhood bed at home days later, I never felt more alone. I went from lying in bed with someone to cuddling my stuffed animal solo underneath my sheets.

The first few days after I was ghosted were extremely difficult. The situation was agonizing because my anxiety was triggered by his abrupt absence. I would close my eyes, sit in silence, and ruminate over what went wrong. I ran every detail through my mind hundreds of times. It was unproductive. I couldn't go about my day without stopping to think about what happened. It felt like I would never be satisfied until I had an answer. I knew we weren't going to date. I knew where I stood emotionally. The ambiguity surrounding the bait and switch is what left me stuck in the past.

I considered confronting him about the situation over the phone, but I ultimately decided to hold back. His silence indicated to me that he had nothing to say and that he wouldn't care what I had to say either. I didn't want to be too pushy for the sake of avoiding a fight. Arguments tend to worsen my anxiety. Tensions were already high. Adding fuel to the fire, especially in a situation I was already ruminating over, would make things worse. I worried that I would say the wrong thing, and that forcing him to explain would only leave me more hurt. Besides, what was I even fighting for? We were not in a relationship. I would have been seeking reassurance that he didn't ghost me because I wasn't attractive or I had said something to offend him. Asking him the questions riddled with self-doubt in my head would have fueled my anxiety. It would have shown the anxiety that these questions were real and logical and needed to be addressed when they didn't.

I also know myself and I know that if someone raises their voice in an argument, I crawl back into my shell and my opinion will never be heard. I excessively apologize and beg them not to be upset with me. The argument will become less about us and more about them. I also find myself overanalyzing the situation aloud. I talk in circles and raise issues that don't need to be raised. Arguments make me feel fragile and unstable. They leave an even deeper pit in my stomach than the one that was there to begin with. In this case, I decided it was best to avoid any further interaction with him.

When I look back at our time together, a lot of it is blurry. I close my eyes, and I can recall a few peaks of our weekend. Then, the memories go dark. The highlights quickly transform into nothingness. The pain is palpable. We were not just physically intimate, but emotionally intimate as well. When you open your heart to someone and they leave, it can feel like you're not enough for them. My self-worth was reduced to the size of the vape pen he hid in his pocket all weekend with me. Who gave him the power to make me feel so small and insignificant?

What I'm starting to realize is that this situation was never really about him—it was about me. In all honesty, I don't think I was ever even attracted to him. I was attracted to the way he made me feel: sexy, self-confident, and witty. I thought I was chasing him, but in reality, I was chasing that feeling. It was like a drug. Whenever I was around him, I liked myself. I opened up a new side of me, not because of the person he was, but because he was someone I knew well and felt comfortable around. The stakes were low. It was never about the guy running away. It was about a feeling of self-confidence I was addicted to suddenly being snatched from under me. He never had the power to make me feel sad, because he was never the one who made me happy. The euphoria came from within.

I realized that I don't necessarily need to talk to him to find closure. It's common to believe reassurance will lead to recovery, but I know myself well, and I know my anxiety will never be satisfied. I'm learning how to center myself without leaning too heavily on anyone else. Mastering your mind is a superpower. Follow your breath inward. You already know what's best for you. I seek closure through my own means. I move forward and try my best not to look back. This situation taught me just how much I value intimacy. I knew that the next person I wanted to give my body to would be someone I was positive about, someone I knew wouldn't leave.

As for the anxiety and mental rumination, I'm proud of myself for being able to identify it. I can look back at that evening and separate genuine emotion from anxiety. Of course, I'm hurt. Who wouldn't be if the man they chose to be intimate with unexpectedly disappeared? But I'm well aware that searching for answers will lead nowhere. Why waste time thinking about something you can't change when the possibility for something greater lies ahead?

SELF-CARE CORNER:

PROTECT YOUR PEACE

You are going to be met with situations in life that challenge your boundaries. A friend might criticize you behind your back. A date might use you solely for his own physical pleasure. A parent might hold you back from embracing your true identity. This goes for everyone, but especially if you suffer from a mental health disorder: it's essential to protect your emotional and physical well-being.

Every day, you must wake up and choose you. You know yourself better than anyone. You know where your line is and when it's crossed. Be patient with yourself and others, but also don't feel like you have to stay in situations that put your mental or physical health at risk. There's a difference between embracing discomfort and being unsafe. Doing things that push you outside your comfort zone is fine and encouraged, but when you feel like it's going to hinder your well-being, it might be time to step away.

There are active ways to protect your peace. First, become conscious of your triggers. If a particular person or topic causes you anxiety, set your boundaries. Cutting negative people out of your life doesn't make you a bad person. It means you're smart and self-aware. Embrace people who make you feel good about yourself rather than tear you down. Those who cheer you on instead of criticizing your successes are worth holding onto.

Don't be afraid to communicate your desires. If you're craving a night on the couch instead of going out with friends, speak up. If a loved one isn't hearing you, express how you feel unapologetically. Owning who you are from the inside out is the only way to protect your peace. Trust your gut, and always put yourself first.

CHAPTER 5

GRIEF

I've never lost anyone as a young adult. Boyfriends? Sure. Keys? Definitely. But family members? And for good? Never. My grandpa and great grandma passed away when I was a child. Although tragic for my parents, I don't remember it, or them, well. I didn't understand what loss meant back then. There's no rule book on how to handle grief and the anxiety that may accompany it. That's why when it hit, I was not prepared.

My grandma Gaga passed away recently. It was a domino effect: first her legs, then her lungs, then her heart. I watched the light leave her eyes, the energy fade from her voice. In her final days, she wasn't the same upbeat person who called me every night to find out "what's doin'?" She wasn't the grandma who would press me for every detail of my dates or beg for a full recap of my school day. As I witnessed her lying on her hospital bed, she looked lifeless and empty.

Gaga was always full of light. She called me twice a day, and my mom at least five times. In elementary and middle school, we spoke every night while I was in the shower, what we named a "potty call." I would place the phone outside the shower door, on the edge of the sink, and shout over the running water while telling her about my classes. As a former principal, she was fascinated by my course curriculums. I would send her an email about every "A" I received.

As time went on, she started to stumble verbally and physically, whether over words or her own two feet. She snapped sporadically out of frustration—something my mom often called the "Jekyll and Hyde" effect. She blamed my mom for her current situation—everything from her uncomfortable corner chair in the emergency room to her lukewarm water bottle to her buckling legs. "It's all your fault," she said. The sad thing is, as my mom heard the passion in my grandma's words and saw the anger in her eyes, she believed her. It wasn't fair. My mom was working so hard to make her happy. She did not deserve to feel rejected.

No matter how much I tried to tell my mom she did a good job taking care of my grandma, it didn't seem to register. I couldn't imagine what she was going through: the endless hospital calls, midnight jitters, paperwork, and screaming matches with her sister. I had never seen her anxiety that severe. I told her she's my superwoman, my hero, my everything. But all she saw was her mom, who was once her everything as well, slipping away.

When someone you love is deteriorating, what is there to do? Besides providing a hug and a shoulder to cry on, not much. I presented my mom with a Dammit Doll to slam on the table. "You can't control the situations, but you can control your reaction," I said, encouraging her to take her anger out on the toy. She refused. So we sat in silence, crying and holding each other. I told her I wasn't letting go until I knew she was okay. In that moment, she was not okay, and as long as she wasn't, neither was I.

In taking care of my mom, I wasn't really able to focus on myself or process what happened: my grandma is gone. My anxiety is breaking through as I cope with grief. Given my history with intrusive thoughts about death and suicide, I wasn't sure what to expect from attending a funeral. I worried that the intense emotions I faced and conquered back in 2020 would resurface at the funeral home and cemetery. Would the candles, dark clothing, and prayers ignite my intrusive thoughts?

I willingly placed myself in situations where I could be triggered. I even challenged myself to write the eulogy to take the weight off my mom and pay tribute to my grandma. I knew how difficult it was for my mom, so I assumed the responsibility in her place. She was well aware that my intrusive thoughts might be set off. "Are you sure?" she asked in tears. I had watched her cycle through boxes of tissues over the past week. I was positive. This was something I wanted to do, not just for my grandma, but for my mom as well.

Surprisingly, the mental rumination over what could happen was worse than what actually happened. As I delivered my grandma's eulogy, I was numb. I didn't even shed a tear. I felt like a robot, merely going through the motions. After the funeral, I went home and hopped on my bike for an hour and a half. It was business as usual. I was proud of how I handled the service. It spoke to how much work I put into my mental health and how far I had come in my anxiety journey. But when grief and anxiety intertwine, it's complicated. Emotions strike when you least expect them.

The other night, I cried for the first time since she passed. My grandma came to me in one of my dreams to tell me she missed me, and I woke up in the middle of the night hysterical. I wanted the dream to continue so I could spend more time with her, but my anxiety shot me awake. My mom ran inside my room to console me as I hyperventilated. This wasn't the first dream I'd had about my grandma. The anxiety was persistent. I felt on edge and out of control both in my sleep and when I woke up. I had ignored the abnormal behavior until one evening when it came to a head. "I can't believe I'll never see her again," I cried. "I don't know how I can go on without her."

Now that she's gone, I can't pick up the phone and call her to share my successes or ask for advice. It breaks my heart, and my mom's as well, that she won't be at my college graduation. It crushes me that she won't be able to hold my book in her hands. But I'm at peace knowing that she was so proud of me. She told me consistently that I was her pride and joy, and that she loved me more than anything. She passed knowing that her daughter raised me to be a strong woman, daughter, and future wife and mother. It's not worth it to ruminate over what's missing because her legacy is alive and strong.

When I went to the hospital to say goodbye to her, I shut the curtain so we could be alone. Yet I found myself at a loss for words. I just kept repeating "We're all here. I love you," over and over again. She mumbled "I love you, too" and blew me a kiss.

I told her over the phone that everything was going to be okay, and she said "okay." After she passed, I felt like a fraud. She wasn't with us anymore, so how could she be okay? Then, I tried to place myself inside of her mind. Gaga cared about her family so much. When I said everything was going to be okay, she most definitely was thinking about me, my mom, my aunt, and my dad. I didn't know it at the time, but my words were a pledge that we would be okay without her. We would not just survive but thrive. As I've been telling my mom, we will work through this together, one step at a time.

While we try to navigate our way through what comes next, I'm practicing patience with both myself and my mom. Dealing with grief is difficult and complex, especially for someone with anxiety. I'm aware of the intense emotions I may experience, and I accept them. Experiencing loss is inevitable as you mature. No one lives forever.

When my grandma was fading, she was difficult to talk to over the phone. She seemed disengaged from the conversation when really, she just had a hard time following what I was saying. It wasn't her fault. Because she was declining, our chats weren't as rich as they used to be. I would make phone calls quick and simple. Our one-hour conversations turned into brief check-ins that lasted five minutes or less. Looking back now, I think part of me knew her time was coming, and hearing her struggle with words was too difficult to bear.

I ruminate over the fact that I didn't spend as much time on the phone with her as I could have in her final few months. She stayed at home all day. I could've called her so much more. She would've loved it. But I never did. It breaks my heart that I didn't take advantage of what I had when I had it. Now, I'll never have it again. It makes me anxious to think about how I dreaded phone calls with her in the end because of how disengaged she was. I feel like a bad person. I should have empathized more. I should have told her how much I loved her more.

I've learned that with anxiety, "shoulds" and "shouldn'ts" are the enemy. It's easy to look at any situation and think about how you could have acted differently. But everything happens for a reason. Everyone who loses someone they love wishes for more time with them. It's never enough. As much as I wanted to call her more in the end, she just wasn't the same, and it hurt to hear her voice. She wouldn't want me to remember her that way. Admitting that doesn't make me a bad person, nor does it mean I loved her any less.

Gaga knew how much I loved her. I would conclude every phone call with a kiss and an "I love you" up until the last time we spoke. It's not her forgiveness I'm seeking for shortening our calls—it's mine. I'm still working on it, but the more I think about the hugs I enveloped her in, the closer I am to getting there.

The most important thing I've realized while grieving is to never take anyone for granted. When someone dies, it's natural to wish for more: one more hug, one more kiss, one more phone conversation. But instead of getting stuck in the past, I savor the present. I pull my mom closer. I squeeze her hand tighter. I love her more than I ever have before.

Gaga is my first great love lost. There's no timeline as to when you finally move forward after someone close to you passes. In fact, trying to expedite the process may put you at risk of pushing down emotions that might resurface later. I allow myself to feel each stage of grief in its entirety. I let the tears flow. I give myself time and space to reminisce. And if I'm angry, I'll have the Dammit Doll ready and waiting, just in case my mom or I ever decide to use it. We're in this together.

SELF-CARE CORNER:

PRACTICE PATIENCE

Anxiety isn't a one-and-done type of thing. Whether you like it or not, it can be a long battle. It's understandable to want to rush to get better so that your symptoms subside. There's no medal at the end of the race to reward you if your anxiety goes away. The real prize is finding peace in the fact that it's okay to live with it. When you practice patience with yourself, you will eventually find comfort in discomfort.

Practicing patience means showing yourself grace, particularly when you're feeling low. It means accepting situations that are out of your hands. It means allowing yourself to cry, to fail, and to fail again. Sometimes, you don't even know why you're crying. Learning how to cope with anxiety takes time. Just because you've been fighting for years and it's still a part of you doesn't make you weak—it makes you a warrior. You will show the most progress when you learn how to pick yourself up and keep trying. Moving past your anxiety is not about waiting for the moment you are never anxious again. The real growth is when you feel anxious and go forth anyway. Your mind may be screaming, but your spirit roars loader.

Of course, you have to put in the work. Being patient doesn't mean being passive. You can enlist a therapist, counselor, family member, friend or helpline for support. You can assemble a toolkit of tactics to dig into when your anxiety arises. You can carve out time in your schedule for self-care as if it's a work appointment. If you dedicate yourself to bettering your mental health, you're already on the right path, and your mood may improve without you even realizing.

CHAPTER 6

IN-BETWEEN

I feel like I'm in an in-between phase right now. Not bad, but not great either. Those with anxiety often highlight high-intensity episodes, moments of excruciating fear and panic. But what about the in-between moments? It feels like you're coasting, but not really. Like watching a calm ocean with a voice in the back of your head telling you a wave might come and sweep you away without warning. I can never *not* be anxious, because even when my intrusive thoughts are gone, I'm anxious about being anxious. I'm on edge and worried that something might trigger me. And guess what? When you look for anxiety, you will find it. If you tell yourself something's going to make you anxious, you'll be in your head searching for a reason to panic, whether you want to or not. Why look for anxiety, I ask myself, when you want so badly to get rid of it?

Sometimes, I feel like being anxious is my baseline. If I wake up in the morning and don't have a sense of self-doubt, I feel abnormal. I have spent so many moments wallowing in anxiety, it has become a blanket of sorts for me. If I enjoy myself for an hour when I'm out running, for example, I find myself immediately checking for my anxiety when I come off the high. It's as if my brain is saying, "Woah, you actually feel good? That can't be right." I'm constantly waiting for something to go wrong.

Anxiety goes through phases. One day, you feel like you're on top of the world, and the next, you can't get out of bed. Life is a balance. Negativity can only weigh you down for so long before you go back to balance, and soon enough, positivity will take its turn. My friends tell me I deserve inner peace. Is that even possible? When I wake up in the morning with intense anxiety (it's always worse when the sun comes up), I have a hard time believing it'll get better.

I'm prone to anxious dreams that don't wake me up in the middle of the night but have a profound effect on me in the morning. Sometimes, when my alarm rings, I wake up with my heart pounding and my sheets drenched in sweat. I typically recall every detail of the dream at the root of these anxiety symptoms.

Today was no different. For as long as I can remember, I've had the same recurring anxious dream: I'm in my high school, raising my hand in English class, when

I smell gas. Then, I notice fire through the window. The fire alarm goes off, and students and teachers rush down five flights of stairs. I exit out the back staircase and sprint as far from the building as possible. When I'm about an avenue away, I witness my high school being blown up by terrorists. I don't have my phone, so I just keep running home for miles, worried about what my mom will think when she hears about the terrorist attack on the news.

Just because you have a disturbing dream doesn't mean it's going to come to fruition. Most of the time, my dreams signify my underlying generalized anxiety disorder. Your brain is free to roam in waking life, and it does the same when you're asleep. Dreams can be complete nonsense. They're not supposed to be obsessed over when you wake up.

Still, it's difficult for me not to try to assign some meaning to my dreams, particularly when they're distressing. I've had the terrorist attack dream repeatedly, so I've come to terms with the fact that it's a glaring symbol of my anxiety. Just as I have intrusive thoughts during waking hours, I sometimes experience intrusive dreams as well. The content is similar—sometimes even more troubling. I wake up shaken, considering why my brain might be having unsettling thoughts on a subconscious level. Are there hidden themes I've been avoiding in my waking life? Should I be concerned that my brain is wandering wildly when I'm asleep? Any feelings or memories I push away in daily life tend to emerge while I sleep so I can process them.

Dreams do not necessarily represent desires. Intrusive dreams and intrusive thoughts function similarly in that manner. They can be vivid, perturbing, and persistent. They can be against your beliefs and not align with the core of who you are. Let's say you have an anxious dream about an ex, even when you're in a loving and happy relationship. Anxiety targets your values, even when you're sleeping. This dream may only demonstrate that you value loyalty and trust in your relationship. Intrusive dreams also don't necessarily have an explicit trigger. It's very possible that you can have a great day and anxious sleep that evening. You simply may be having more vivid dreams because you're tired, which makes REM sleep deeper and more intense.

Intrusive thoughts during the day can be more easily controlled through meditation, movement, and work. With intrusive dreams, it's more difficult to escape. When you're stuck in an unconscious state, it's hard to shake yourself awake and realize it's not your reality. I usually have a hard time waking myself up from a bad dream and rely on my morning alarm to do so.

Most frustrating of all is when my OCD extends beyond sleep and lasts throughout the day. I know the feeling will pass eventually, but when my brain is loud, it's hard to listen to logic. My surroundings become blurry, and I feel deper-sonalized. I can't see clearly. Intrusive thoughts pop up at random times, in random places, when I'm just trying to exist. They can be in the form of commands. For example, "you should hurt your dog!" or "slice your finger off!" The thoughts can be uncomfortable or disturbing, particularly if they are of a sexual or destructive nature that is unin-vited. OCD also comes in the form of a question—rather, a tornado of questions. The questions may be simple, but they sting. They're unorthodox and overwhelming. What if my house catches on fire? What if that car rounding the corner hits me? How will people remember me when I die? Thoughts are thoughts. It's okay to let your mind wander. But for someone with OCD, those "what if" thoughts can become highly distressing and debilitating. They bring you out of your body and into your head, where you attempt to disprove them. Even when you think you've won by finding the logic you were searching for, the feel-ing is temporary. Before long, another question arises that brings you back to where you started. The cycle is endless.

Anxiety hits unexpectedly. As much as I anticipate anxious moments, each one still takes my breath away. In these moments, nothing feels stable. Everything feels fleeting. I feel unsure of everything and everyone around me—how do they feel about me? How do I feel about them? Am I doing everything "right" in my life? I'm not my usual bubbly self. I feel alone, yet easily irritable when around other people. It's confusing. I don't know whether to sit in it solo or surround myself with others.

Most of the time, I'm fixated on a specific intrusive thought, but that's not always the case. Sometimes, the feeling is more broad and generalized. Every intrusive thought I've ever had runs through my head on repeat, and I have an all-consuming feeling of guilt and anxiety.

If you struggle with guilt as well, think back to the first time you ever felt guilty. One of the greatest sources of guilt from my childhood was quitting dance after 14 years. I worked so hard to perfect this craft, only to walk away from it. I felt like a disappointment to myself and my family, who spent considerable time and money funding classes and recital costumes. I stepped away from ballet over five years ago, but oddly enough, when I feel guilty over my intrusive thoughts, I recognize that it's a similar feeling. The more I talk to my therapist about my lingering emotions surrounding my exit from dance, the better equipped I feel dealing with my guilt. All this goes to say, don't be afraid to trace back those intense emotions and see where they might be coming from.

Separating thought from feeling also helps in anxious moments. Feeling guilty doesn't necessarily mean my thoughts are true. They're not 'good' or 'bad.' They're just words inside my mind with no meaning. The feelings—

guilt, dread, shame—are because of the anxiety disorder, not because the intrusive thoughts hold truth. Defusion helps desensitize you to your thoughts. The goal is to realize that disturbing thoughts may be annoying, but they're not dangerous.

THERAPIST'S COUCH:

COGNITIVE DEFUSION

According to Mindie Barnett,
LAC, Associate Therapist

Cognitive defusion is a technique used in Acceptance and Commitment Therapy, which helps people separate themselves from thoughts causing them discomfort. The practice involves creating a space between the person and their thoughts and feelings, which helps them become more aware of their overall thinking process. An example of this is envisioning one's thoughts in a bubble above them. This enables the person to become more mindful of their thoughts and also maintain the ability to separate themselves from difficult thoughts and feelings.

I've never been into meditation, but mindfulness is an effective technique to defuse anxiety. I picture my anxiety as a ball of fire in my brain. It's bright. It's piping hot, too hot to touch. Once I visualize the anxiety as fire, I realize that it's just energy. I close my eyes and imagine the ball of fire moving through my body: into my arms, my legs, my stomach. I try to feel the fire on whichever part of my body I'm focusing on. I'm not pushing the fire away per se, but I'm showing my brain that it's fully in my command.

Visualization can be extremely beneficial. Sometimes, to refocus myself, I close my eyes and transport to somewhere else. It's like a game. I'll ask myself, *what does your dream future look like?* Or, *when you think about your childhood, where does your mind go?* Then, I'll describe out loud what I see: my bed, the trees outside the window, the stuffed animal sitting on my dresser. Where am I? Who's with me? What do my surroundings smell like? What do I hear? It's fun to think of new and exciting questions that grant my brain freedom to roam.

Sometimes, I'll even let a loved one in on the activity and picture the world they're describing as they speak. Talking about my anxiety openly and casually with a loved one revives me. It helps normalize the intrusive thoughts and reminds me that even though my brain might be aflame, in reality, everything is okay.

It can be hard to find people to confide in about anxiety because of the stigma. Many people will misunderstand your feelings. Trust me, I know. It took years for me to find people to open up to. It's worth the effort when you gather a team that supports you and understands when you're at a low point. They're the ones who will stick around through it all—the highs, the lows, and the in-between.

SELF-CARE CORNER:

VISUALIZATION

I'll be the first to admit it: I hate meditation. Being alone with my thoughts makes me antsy. I'm someone who thrives off of movement and exercise. Standing still and listening to my breath when all I want to do is run free drives me mad. I don't think I'll ever become a yogi, but some techniques used in yoga and meditation have been helpful in coping with my anxiety.

It's amazing what the mind can do to calm the body if you really focus. Try picturing anxiety as something tangible, like a storm cloud or a raging flame you need to extinguish. You can get creative, even though it might feel silly sometimes. Putting a picture to the emotion helps to desensitize. It makes the anxiety seem like less of a burden and more of something you can tackle head on. You may not be able to control your intrusive thoughts, but you can control your reaction to them.

My favorite type of visualization is picturing my anxiety dissipating as I watch it float away on a cloud. Some days, I walk it to a chair at the back of my head. I also love picturing something I'm looking forward to in the future. I imagine what it would look like if I achieved one of my goals. What's the scene? What do I see, hear, and smell around me? I usually take my mind to the marathon finish line. There's confetti showering down from the sky, cheers from every angle, and a heavy medal strung around my neck. Spend time soaking in the moment, and allow yourself to enjoy the possibility of it happening. The imagery takes me out of my head and into my heart as I'm reminded of what I'm most passionate about.

You can also use visualization to picture yourself in a safe space. Close your eyes and take yourself to your happy place. Is it a beach? An amusement park? The street you grew up on? A field of flowers? Engage your five senses while exploring your imagination. The mere thought of something beautiful or joyful can remind you why life is worth living.

CHAPTER 7
WEAK

I may be a marathon runner, but today, I feel anything but strong. I may be an author, but right now, I don't feel inspired. When the present and future are so bright, sometimes, I get burned. The spotlight and success feel too good to be true.

Last week's book launch for *My Real-Life Rom-Com* was the best week of my life, a culmination of hard work and progress when it comes to my mental health. I mention my anxiety in the last chapter of *Rom-Com*, which focuses on finding self-love. The majority of news anchors and interviewers who spoke to me about the book asked for my advice about how to beat anxiety and learn to love yourself. But it makes me feel uncertain: who am I to be preaching about how others can help their anxiety when I'm sitting here alone, teary-eyed and wondering how to help myself?

Intrusive thoughts are sticky, strange and hard to understand. Even though I am fully aware they're false, merely a result of my anxiety disorder, I still struggle. Perhaps most troubling is when I seek reassurance from others. I confess intrusive thoughts that mean nothing, but that I feel compelled to say aloud to "double-check" that nobody else cares. Here's the kicker: oversharing is problematic when it becomes a pattern. Our minds are for us and us only. Every thought that crosses your mind does not need to be shared. Intrusive thoughts in particular are not meant to be blurted out. They're called "garbage thoughts" for a reason. And sometimes, when they are confessed, they can really hurt someone. It's not the intrusive thought itself that's harmful—it's the act of sharing it.

You'd think I'd know better at this point, but everyone makes mistakes. It's hard to admit weakness. This month, I'm going to be greeting readers on my book tour. People expect me to be the upbeat personality they see on their television screens and TikTok "For You" pages. I'm supposed to be the girl who is always smiling. That's the Carrie that people see on the outside: happy, successful, and exuberant. I love smiling. But I'll admit, I haven't genuinely smiled or laughed in at least a week. All I feel right now is scared—scared of losing myself, and scared of losing the people I love when I show this anxious side of myself. I can't be cheerful all the time. This earthquake of emotions feels impossible to bear.

I want to be vulnerable, to open up to friends and family about my anxiety and obsessive thoughts, but I don't want to be a burden. I don't want to annoy them to the point where I push them away. I read online that others can relate, but what I really crave is reassurance from my loved ones. It's hard for them to understand. "I thought OCD was about everything being perfect and super clean," my best friend once told me. "Oh, you have OCD, so you must be really organized," another friend said. The majority of my OCD is centered around thought rumination. It has nothing to do with cleanliness or organization. My friends have no idea how difficult it can be—they only know what they've seen or read in media. For example, Sheldon in *The Big Bang Theory* needing to knock three times, which is merely laughed off. There's more to OCD than what you see on the screen.

THERAPIST'S COUCH:

OCD VS. OCPD

*According to Nathan Peterson, OCD Therapist
and Licensed Clinical Social Worker*

OCPD is commonly misdiagnosed as OCD. Although Obsessive-Compulsive Disorder (OCD) and Obsessive-Compulsive Personality Disorder (OCPD) might seem similar, understanding the differences is important so people can get the support they need.

OCD is a mental health condition centered around obsessive thoughts and compulsions. Someone with OCD may find it difficult to stop thinking about certain things and end up performing the same actions repeatedly to try to feel better. For example, checking multiple times to see if the stove is off or ruminating over past conversations to ensure they didn't say anything "wrong." Those with OCD don't want to perform these compulsions, but they can't help it.

OCPD is more about being highly attentive to detail and order. Someone with OCPD likes

everything done in a specific way. This is a personality disorder focused on perfectionism and control. They lack flexibility in their actions and are
extremely rigid in their routine.

The main difference between OCD and OCPD
is how people feel about their thoughts. If you have
OCD, you don't like your thoughts because they
don't align with what you really believe. But with
OCPD, your thoughts match your beliefs, and you
think everyone else should do things your way, too.

Symptoms of OCD include extreme worrying, double-checking, and persistent intrusive
thoughts. OCPD symptoms might involve being
strict about forming rules or always wanting to do
things yourself.

Although I wish my friends and family could help,
you can't expect everyone to be on the same page. Besides,
OCD feeds off of reassurance. It's never fully satisfied,
and it often feels like you're in a loop, thinking about
and confessing the same thought until you "feel better."
That process is like filling a cup with a hole in it—simply ineffective. If I confess, I feel ashamed. If I hold my
intrusive thoughts in, OCD makes me feel like I'm being

dishonest and lying to myself and those around me. I can't win.

My mom always steps in with logic. She'll ask me why I'm feeling anxious even when I have no explanation. She'll try to come up with her own "why" the intrusive thought was there in the first place. Trying to figure out why a certain intrusive thought arose is counterproductive. It takes you out of reality and into your imagination. There's no need to look so deeply into a thought when that's all it is—a thought. Furthermore, it's a thought you don't agree with. Although I understand her motherly instinct to solve the problem, attempting to untangle my anxiety is like taking on a ten-foot bully. Her advice doesn't make a dent.

I've tried to be proactive in alleviating my anxiety. I sit with it in the back of my brain while trying to go about my day. But OCD always fires back with the hard questions: how do you know? Are you positive you don't agree with these thoughts? Just when I think I've answered all the questions, my brain finds a way to spit out more. The cycle is agonizing. I've suffered through several physical anxiety attacks this month—shaky hands, nausea, dizziness and all.

It took tough love from the person I love most to garner the courage to write about my emotions, to own how I'm feeling without keeping it all bottled inside my head.

He said to fight for myself. He told me that he can support me as much as I need, but he can't pull me out of it—only I can do that. I could see the frustration in his eyes as he stared past me while uttering those words. I almost sensed shame, as if he knew I was better than that. The girl who went on TV talking about her anxiety is much stronger than the girl who sat there telling the same old story about her intrusive thoughts for the fourth day in a row. She knows better.

My therapist would tell me that trying to figure out why my intrusive thoughts are there is a waste of time. Everyone occasionally has thoughts they don't agree with. For people with OCD, these thoughts can consume you. Why do they come up in the first place? It's just par for course with an anxiety disorder. The less you check to see if the thoughts are there, the better you'll feel. It's not fair, I know. You're supposed to say when they pop up, "hi, you're just anxiety." Easier said than done when you're stuck in an obsessive thought loop.

Thoughts are not facts. Close your eyes and think to yourself that the sky is purple or that snow is hot. The words your brain tells you aren't necessarily true. There is no need to stop an intrusive thought or deny that it exists. The more you push back, the more incessant the thought becomes. It may live rent free in your mind, but that doesn't mean you have to feed it. Become a witness, not a worrier. Do not engage. Instead, direct your energy toward something more productive, even if it feels like you're forcing yourself to move forward. Journaling helps, like what I'm doing right now. It took me a few days to get here, though. Recentering yourself can be difficult. It takes time.

As I write, I'm reminded of something tucked away that a therapist told me a while back: intrusive thoughts are ego-dystonic. It is a scientifically proven fact that your intrusive thoughts are opposite of who you are and what you believe. Those with violent intrusive thoughts may actually value living a beautiful life. Those with intrusive thoughts about hurting their family may actually be concerned about their loved ones' safety. Intrusive thoughts attack the people and things you love most in the world. You know the thoughts aren't real or true because they scare you. They are unwelcome thoughts. You don't like them, and they don't align with who you are. If the thoughts were valid or relevant, you wouldn't necessarily be so eager to expel them from your brain.

THERAPIST'S COUCH:

EGO–DYSTONIC

According to Kimberley Quinlan,
LMFT, Anxiety and OCD Therapist

"Ego-dystonic" is a psychological term used to describe thoughts, impulses, and behaviors that are against an individual's self-perception, values, and beliefs. When something is ego-dystonic, it feels foreign, distressing, and inconsistent with one's values and self-image. This causes significant internal conflict, anxiety, and discomfort.

The concept of something being ego-dystonic is crucial in understanding certain mental health conditions, particularly OCD. In OCD, the intrusive thoughts or compulsive behaviors are often ego-dystonic. An individual with OCD might have repetitive, distressing thoughts about causing harm to others, despite having no desire to act on these thoughts and finding them repugnant. This discord between the thoughts and the person's values can lead to severe anxiety and distress.

In contrast, the term "ego-syntonic" refers to thoughts and behaviors that are consistent with the individual's self-perception and values and do not cause internal conflict. Understanding whether a thought or behavior is ego-dystonic or ego-syntonic is important in both diagnosis and treatment. When a therapist recognizes that a patient's distress stems from ego-dystonic thoughts, they can tailor interventions to address their intrusive thoughts.

Intrusive thoughts are often misunderstood, and they have been for a long time. Sigmund Freud, the founder of psychoanalysis, considered individuals with OCD to be those who had "taboo desires" within the realm of normal society. I believe this early musing is fundamentally wrong. Rendering OCD thoughts as "taboo desires" grants them a sense of realness. They are anything but a "desire," no matter what OCD tries to convince us.

It's natural to play off any unwelcome thought as "intrusive." For someone with OCD, these thoughts are not just uninvited, but they can be highly upsetting and contrary to the core of who they are. Wanting ice cream in the middle of the night is not an intrusive thought (even though you might feel guilty about it, it's something you actually desire). Nor is thinking about food in the middle of a funeral (the thought may be involuntary, but it isn't against your values or beliefs).

Intrusive thoughts are harder to handle and generally much more bothersome. When they creep in, and you're eager to restore balance, just think about the science. Don't treat it like an escape thought—something you repeat to yourself compulsively when the intrusion sets in—but let this sink in: intrusive thoughts are fundamentally opposite from reality. Let that bring you some peace. It took me about thirty minutes of journaling, but I reached that conclusion myself. I guess the ability was inside me all along.

SELF-CARE CORNER:

JOURNALING

Journaling your feelings is therapeutic—and I'm not just saying that because I'm a writer. Since I was little, I've kept a diary. Writing has helped me find closure with certain situations and brought me closer to myself. I leave each session with a stronger sense of who I am. Writing is home for me. I feel most like myself with a pen and paper in hand.

The number one reason I hear people don't like to write is because they lack inspiration. They tell me they don't know what to write about or they're not sure where to start. When it comes to writing about yourself, I don't buy that excuse. I'll be blunt: maybe you're just scared. Maybe you're shying away from the unknown that will reveal itself when words start flowing on the page. But breaking through that fear is where you will see the most growth. When you're finally honest about your emotions with yourself, you start to accept them. They become a lot less scary when they're out of your mind and staring back at you on the paper. After all, they're just words.

Journaling provides the privacy to slow down and organize your thoughts. For me, cozying up on the couch with a diary is calming. It's a safe space that encourages me to open up to myself and identify thought patterns and behaviors. There's freedom in self-awareness. The more you know who you are, the less power anxiety holds over you.

CHAPTER 8
FEAR

I'm scared. Why is it that every single morning, like clockwork, the first thing I feel is fear? I'm tired of being scared—scared of myself, scared of my thoughts, scared this will never get better. No matter how many intrusive thoughts I have, each one feels like the first. Each one is darker and more disturbing than the previous one. Just when I think it can't get any worse, it does. As I sit here alone in my bedroom, swallowing my tears while writing, I'll admit it's really hard. Although writing is therapeutic for me, when it comes to my mental health, it simultaneously feels like an exposure.

I go about my day—working out, going to college, hanging out with friends—and act like my intrusive thoughts aren't there when they are. They always are. I'm constantly pretending I'm okay when deep down, I'm not. I mean, I suppose I am, but anxiety can make it feel like the world is ending. I can engage in an exciting activity or achieve an accomplishment and still feel like I'm hurting for no reason.

I woke up this morning feeling decent—never good, always decent. I snoozed my alarm but instantly regretted it, because during those nine extra minutes of shut-eye, I had an intrusive dream. My alarm went off again and my heart started pounding because I knew this thought would be stubborn. I've only been awake for three hours today, but I'm upset, frustrated, and depersonalized. No matter how much I want to live in the moment—to enjoy my upcoming lunch with a friend, to look forward to the surprise date I planned for my boyfriend tonight—I can't.

Just like that, my tears are back. They're still being swallowed. I've convinced myself that a full-on cry means something is really wrong. It means that OCD has the power. It won today. And that's not something I want or need to acknowledge.

As my hands hover (okay, tremble) over my computer, I'm still scared. There's a sense of shame and guilt attached to the fact that intrusive thoughts can linger, so much so that I lose track of how much time it's been. Intrusive thoughts seem to flow in a circular motion. They're not a one-and-done type of thing. I was stuck on the same intrusive thought for a few weeks about three months ago. I thought it was never going to let up until one day,

I got so frustrated and angry, it disappeared. I strongly disagreed with the thought from the start, but weeks in, I wasn't just upset to be living with it, I was furious. So it went away. My brain began to obsess over a different intrusive thought—also troubling, but more tolerable than the former.

Fast forward to now: after battling a slew of different intrusive thoughts over the past few months, the same one from before is back. It's as if my brain were so annoyed that I conquered all these thoughts, it said, "Let's give Carrie another challenge. Let's bring back the worst thought all over again to see how she handles it this time around." I guess I'm handling it better so far. I'm not having a full-blown panic attack. But I'm disturbed, and I'm scared as to why the thought is still there. The longer a thought remains, the more you start to wonder if it's true. I know it's not *actually* true, but that's OCD's job: to make you question who you are, what you love, who you love, and what you value. I can identify my current thought pattern as OCD because of the strong urge I have to confess my thought. If the thought were true, I wouldn't be so inclined to say it aloud.

I'm more scared of my own mind than I am of anything and anyone that comes into my life. The nonsense that enters my brain is more difficult to deal with than any other challenge in the outside world. I went skydiving recently and hardly had any nerves. Jumping out of an airplane at 120 miles per hour was nothing compared to the mental battle I endure every day.

What am I even battling? Lies? Nonsense? It's not like I'm facing an actual threat, but the intruder in my brain feels real, like a burglar entering my house unannounced to steal all my valuables. Intrusive thoughts function similarly: they are the intruder. They enter my brain without warning to try to steal the joy from my everyday life. The result: feeling empty and helpless. When those "valuables" are taken from my brain, a void is left that feels like it's never going to be filled. It doesn't matter how much love and positivity I'm showered with—somehow, it feels like something is missing.

My twenty-first birthday just passed, and the celebration was memorable—not in a good way. It had all the potential to be special. My boyfriend and best friend planned a "surprise" sushi dinner in Los Angeles with a bunch of friends. I was aware of what was happening, but I didn't know who was going to be there. All the friends who came were people I hadn't seen for at least a year or two. We spent most of our time playing catch-up at the table.

After dinner, everyone went home, except for a few close friends who went with me to a bar. It was my first time drinking alcohol (not kidding), and I wasn't sure how I was going to react. The drunken state intensified my anxiety. I deal with intrusive thoughts every day, but this was different. They felt stronger, more intense. I couldn't stop crying. Blame the alcohol, but tears don't lie. I was scared. I am scared.

As my surroundings transformed into a dizzying haze, I retreated into my mind. I began to reflect on being twenty-one and what my future would look like. I asked myself, *am I really happy?* That one loaded question caused me to spiral. I began sobbing uncontrollably at the bar. I assumed that as long as I'm having anxiety and intrusive thoughts, I can never be happy and at peace. "I just want to be happy," I cried to my best friend. "I work so hard, but I still feel shitty. It's not fair." She texted my boyfriend to come and help console me. "You're so lucky you have him," she said. "He's the real deal." Her words triggered even more tears. I felt so guilty. It wasn't fair to my boyfriend that he had to deal with this. He put so much effort into planning a fun party, and I wasn't giving him the excited reaction he deserved. I worried he was upset with me, and I also considered the poor impression I was giving the other party guests. I was concerned about myself while constantly worrying what everyone else thought.

"I'm so sorry," I said repeatedly as we left the bar. "I just want to go home." I sat down on the curb and buried my head in my hands. I sent everyone home; it was just my boyfriend and me at this point. He sat beside me and met my eyes. "Are you not happy?" he asked. I didn't know how to answer his question. If being happy meant having no more intrusive thoughts, then no. I wasn't happy. It felt as though I would never be happy. At that moment, I was solely focused on my anxiety. I couldn't see myself living a peaceful life while being burdened by my OCD.

Happiness seems to enter my life unannounced. It manifests through an unexpectedly peaceful walk along the beach or a Netflix show that takes me out of the present, even if just for an hour. There are people and things that make me happy, but I can't force them. I can be at my birthday dinner—the center of attention, showered with love, hugs, and flowers—and still feel anxiety weighing me down.

That doesn't mean I don't *want* to be happy. I'm doing everything I love. I'm writing. I'm running. I have friends and family who love and support me in everything I do. I'm finding that happiness isn't a check mark. It's not something you work toward, achieve, and then just like that, you're happy for the rest of your life. Each day is a series of emotional peaks and valleys. Some moments will be happy while others are stressful, frustrating, and sad. Happiness is not a trophy. No one is happy all the time. True happiness is finding acceptance in emotional undulations.

Part of being happy is accepting the journey. The feeling you get when overcoming a challenge or completing a goal is exhilarating. The climax always feels better than the climb—you just have to be patient. Although anxiety often feels like the world is caving in, in reality, it's not. My family and friends tell me everything is going to be okay. The funny thing is, everything is already okay. It always has been, and it always will be.

The fear of burdening my loved ones when discussing my anxiety weighs on me almost as much as the content of the intrusive thoughts themselves. Particularly when that content relates to them, I engage in a mental tug-of-war of whether to speak up. To confess or not to confess? What would they think if they knew negative thoughts about them were running through my mind? These are people who show me so much affection, and here I am coping with thoughts that cut deep. It's not fair to me, and it's not fair to them.

Getting an intrusive thought about someone you love can be tricky. I find myself pulling them closer to disprove my thoughts and reassure myself that I'm not a bad person. The last thing I want to do is hurt them. But when I keep these thoughts tucked away, it feels like

I'm harboring a nasty secret, and guilt prevents me from being fully present with that person.

Intrusive thoughts hold no truth, so nothing is really "secret." OCD is the liar—not me. What matters most are the things we say to each other that we really mean. Everything else is just garbage. It gets complicated, however, when I have a difficult time differentiating garbage thoughts from truthful ones and begin to confess. I don't know which hurts more: seeing the look on a loved one's face when I tell them the disturbing thought that crossed my mind, or the weight of OCD and the loneliness it causes.

I've been alone in my anxiety since 2020. Sure, my parents have held me and tried to relate. But it feels like nobody understands just how hard it is except me. Everybody is going through something, but everybody is *not* "a little OCD." Not everybody knows what it feels like to wake up every morning afraid. To cry so much during the week that it feels like it should be scheduled into your calendar. To go about your business while feeling like you're never really present. OCD is not an adjective. It can impair you. It's hard and it hurts.

I'm left wondering: How do I deal with it? How do I go on with my life? What I've been told may sound counterintuitive: do nothing. That is the work. Starve your OCD by not giving it any attention. The more you talk back to your intrusive thoughts, the more you're actualizing them. If you spend time ruminating or performing compulsions, you're not teaching your brain a proper lesson. Move on with your life. The more you thrive, the less power you give your OCD.

I know that I'm not supposed to give my intrusive thoughts any energy. It's just noise, I tell myself. But sometimes, I can't help but engage. Sometimes, the thoughts are so loud, they're practically screaming for attention. I can't help but listen. It's frustrating because I'm educated about OCD, yet there are moments when I'm too weak to stand up to it. I'm too vulnerable to tell it to calm down. But maybe that's just the problem—I shouldn't be telling it to calm down. I should just be letting it exist, no matter how loud or quiet it is. If the intrusive thoughts are screaming, let them scream. If they're quiet, don't question why. I like to pretend there's another person in the back of my head fighting OCD for me, an alter ego of sorts, while I'm living in the present.

Present me often dips out of the current moment to check in and make sure everything's okay in anxiety world. I'm hyper-aware of when my emotions fluctuate; I notice how everything feels great, then terrible, then decent, then depressing. Even though it's hard to believe sometimes, you're stronger than you think. If you just leave your brain alone, it will return to balance naturally. There's no need to be alarmed.

There are moments when I feel hopeful. Like when I come off of a nine-mile run with an adrenaline rush. Or when I write something I'm really proud of. Or after a delicious omakase dinner. Or when my boyfriend smiles at me. Those are the moments I hold onto—small but meaningful.

We're in our minds so much of the time, it's exhausting. What happens if we start to lead with our hearts and souls instead? I often get in my head when things are going well. Why is it so hard to believe we deserve happiness? Instead of questioning peaks of love and light, I wonder what it would feel like to get lost in the magical moments. I wonder what would happen if instead of pushing them away, I fully embraced them.

I'm learning that happiness is a choice, and you can always find things that bring you joy. I run in the park if I want to feel strong. I squeeze my family and friends if I crave a physical connection. I sit on the couch with Honey Bunches of Oats cereal if I need a moment of calm. There is hope everywhere—you just have to be willing to look for it.

SELF-CARE CORNER:

THE FIVE SENSES

You may get lost inside your head when anxiety takes over. Getting caught up in hypotheticals can take you out of the present moment and prevent you from truly living. Engaging your five senses is an easy way to bring yourself back to reality and get grounded. Not only does it give your brain something else to focus on, but it helps you see the world around you in a beautiful light, one that often gets murky when your mind is messing with you.

Start by focusing on your surroundings. Name five things you see around you, and really pay attention to details. Next, move on to five things you feel. If you're walking, it could be your shoes on the pavement or your phone in your hand. If you're in bed, it could be the way your head sinks into the pillow or how your hand brushes the cold sheets. Now focus on five things you can hear. The sounds can be either outdoors or indoors, loud or faint. Identify five things you can smell. This one might be more difficult if you're indoors, but try to focus on any scents emanating from the kitchen or street outside a window. Lastly, name five things you can taste. It might be the leftover Chinese food you just ate or the mint gum you're chewing.

After you've completed this exercise, you'll likely find yourself more relaxed and focused on the present. Remember, practicing mindfulness is not a means of escape from anxiety. It's a way to help you accept anxious thoughts for what they are and gently shift your attention back to reality. Breathe through each step and don't judge yourself if your mind wanders at times. Similar to meditation, if you notice negative thoughts popping up, acknowledge them, let them exist, and slowly bring yourself back.

CHAPTER 9

RESTLESS

No matter where I am or who I'm with, anxiety seems to follow me. I like to think it's conditional, but the reality is, it's not. It's just something I have to live with. I could be sitting on the couch watching football or at the pool on a tropical vacation. The anxiety is there. It's always there.

Currently, I'm staring out at the pool and palm trees in Florida. I just arrived today and expected to feel better. I anticipated that snoozing out in the sunshine would somehow melt away the anxiety. But I couldn't fall asleep. My brain started to wander and think about the same intrusive thoughts and how guilty I feel for having them. A friend told me to explore the thoughts solo, to think about what they are and where they come from. I tried that yesterday in a steam room, and it brought me to a semi-peaceful state. I just tried again by the pool, though, and it feels like I failed. I was so immersed in my own head that I got overwhelmed. I'm several feet away from the water, yet right now, I feel like I'm drowning.

I know I should be grateful for this moment; I'm in a beautiful place on vacation. But when you're enveloped in fear—fear of your own mind, fear of where it wanders and the uninvited thoughts that pop into your head—it's hard to pull yourself out. I wind up just wallowing. I have options laid out in front of me right now to pull myself out. I could read a book. I could walk a few feet and jump into the pool. All I want to do, though, is blow my nose into a beach towel.

In moments of intense anxiety, I rely on my constants to keep me grounded. At home, that's my laptop, my puppy, my cozy Barefoot Dreams blanket. On vacation, these things are out of reach. My OCD makes me want to control every aspect of my life. I never feel more out of sorts than I do when I'm away from home.

It's been that way since I was a little girl. I always hated sleeping away from home because it made me anxious. My heart would pound as I crawled under hotel sheets, and I wouldn't be able to fall asleep for hours. It's ironic, really. You'd think going on vacation would be an escape. You'd assume getting away from everyday anxiety at home would feel liberating. Four days outside of freezing cold New York City to lay by the pool in Florida sounds heavenly. But as I'm sitting here looking out at kids smiling, tossing around a ball in the pool, I can't help but feel disconnected. I don't feel like I'm really here.

When I told my mom how I was feeling, she suggested I start writing in the Notes app on my phone. She thinks every diary entry has some lesson that comes out of it, a resolution of sorts. But I can't come up with one right now. I'm frustrated and scared and sad because I'm anxious and I don't know why. Anxiety doesn't always have a rhyme or reason. It just hits, and it hits painfully hard.

I think back to positive moments I experienced a few months ago, like in Los Angeles on my book tour, and I can't connect the dots on what's changed since then. Honestly, nothing's changed. If anything, life has quieted down since the book tour, and that's a good thing. But since I got home from the last tour stop in Tampa, it's been an avalanche of emotions. It's as if things were going "too well," so something had to give. My anxiety hasn't been this intense since 2020. And that's really scary to admit.

So, what's the solution? I'm told to feel my emotions, not push them down. I'm tired of feeling. I feel too much. But I'd rather feel too much than nothing at all. As humans, we laugh, cry, and immerse ourselves in an emotional rollercoaster fraught with unexpected twists and turns. Feeling the lows also allows us to embrace beautiful highs. Getting my heart broken led me to finding a deep, spiritual connection with a significant other that I could have never imagined. Panic attacks inspired me to take on running, a sport that has grounded me and helped me harness my inner power. Losing my grandma taught me how to love all over again. Out of pain, I found empowerment. My grief inspired me to love stronger and harder and to never take a second with my family for granted. You can be broken and beautiful at the same time. Just because you live with anxiety doesn't mean your life is lost.

Today, I have a hard time figuring out how to do the next right thing. Do I cry? Do I read? Do I cry and read? In moments like these, I tend to feel lonely and lost. What helps is someone hugging me and helping me feel whole again. I rely on others to put the pieces back together for me when I feel too weak to do it myself. I wonder, though, how do I get strong enough to self-soothe?

I assume it's going to take living on my own to develop those skills. I'm generally afraid of being alone with my thoughts. I keep busy and direct my energy toward something productive at all times so I can reside less in my head. Being alone feels like an exposure to me—it's not something I enjoy. But I'm moving into a new apartment solo in January, which I figured is a necessary step in growing up.

I haven't lived alone for more than two weeks at a time. I never spent a summer at sleepaway camp because it was too difficult for me to separate from my home, my family, my routine. When I was twelve years old, I gave it a shot. My parents picked me up not even twenty-four hours after arriving because I called them in tears. They were never the type to make me rough it out if I were by myself and miserable. Looking back now, I wonder if staying would have helped me develop self-sufficiency skills earlier on. Or if staying would have caused me greater anxiety.

It feels like I'm caught in a never-ending sequence of adulting. My looming college graduation, apartment lease and career uncertainties are overwhelming. I assumed the era of "adulting" would conclude after a year of being eighteen, but these past few months leading up to twenty-one have been tough. Time feels heavy, like there's a storm cloud hovering over my life. I can zoom out and see that there's nothing wrong, but somehow, it feels like I'm swept up in a tornado, and nobody understands why I'm so upset. How do I slow down? If it's not a tropical vacation, not the sunshine, then what's the secret? I suppose there is no clear answer, aside from showing myself grace. Forcing myself to go through the motions, to trudge through the chaos, is the only option.

In my opinion, the worst part of anxiety is the way it builds and feels like you're never going to come down. Momentum is a bitch. Emotion is energy. Energy in motion stays in motion. When you work yourself up, it's difficult to get calm. Oftentimes, I get jittery when I start victimizing myself and searching for a "why." Why am I feeling this way? Why am I anxious when nothing is wrong? I've found it's best to stop seeking a "why." When it comes to anxiety, you might not have the answer. You might never have the answer, and that's perfectly fine. It's freeing to release yourself from a need to find a reason why you're anxious. Sometimes, you're anxious because you just are. That's just how your brain is wired. That's a good enough "why."

SELF-CARE CORNER:

LOWER THE STAKES

Taking a passive approach to an intrusive thought is often the best course of action: you don't entertain the thought, merely acknowledge it and move on with your life. However, if you feel that it might be productive, you can explore the thought deeper.

Let me break it down for you. Immersing yourself in an intrusive thought is not to be done when you're busy or out and about. It can become distracting and dangerous. Find a time when you're at home and relaxed before thinking deeply. Make yourself as comfortable as possible. Sit up in your bed, cuddle with your pet, or relax in a warm bubble bath. Once you're settled, identify the intrusive thought and gradually take it to the furthest place it can go. Explore the worst case scenario. Then, respond in a non-alarmist way. Lower the stakes.

Let's say the intrusive thought is that your significant other is cheating on you. Allow yourself to become enveloped in that thought. See it. Feel it. It's going to be hard. It's going to feel uncomfortable. But in the long run, it will help you desensitize yourself. When the intrusive thought arises, turn "what if" into "so what." So what if he cheats? It would be tough in the moment, but you would be grateful you found out. It would only bring you closer to finding the right person for you.

This technique does not work for everyone. Sometimes, exploring the thought does not satisfy OCD and only leaves you to further fixate on it. Work with your therapist to identify the best course of action, particularly if the content of your intrusive thoughts is dark or painful. Either way, the goal is to reframe your intrusive thoughts so that they appear less daunting. The more you approach them with curiosity, the less meaning you begin to prescribe to them.

CHAPTER 10

GROWTH

Nobody prepares you for the moment you realize you're finally growing up. If I'm being logical, I know I've been getting ready for this my whole life. I have my parents to thank: they taught me how to walk to school by myself safely as early as age nine. They emphasized the importance of eating healthy; chicken fingers and pasta were always paired with a new fruit or vegetable. They showed me how to take care of myself and others—how to tell right from wrong, how to balance work and self-care, how to deal with love and loss. And of course, the little things, like how long to keep tuna salad before it spoils, or the difference between a Tide Pod and Cascade pod (hey, they look similar!).

But change is never logical. Change is complex and chaotic. I just moved into my own apartment, and I've never felt more mature. Things have finally settled down in the new place. There are no more movers or contractors drilling. My mom finished helping me organize my Marie Kondo-style closet. My dad set up the Wi-Fi and TV. Now that everyone is gone, I'm alone, and I'm panicking. The silence scares me, as does how quickly time seems to have passed. It feels like just yesterday my parents and I were moving into a new apartment to be closer to my elementary school.

A lot of anxiety stems from anticipatory fear of the future. I'm anxious over becoming anxious, when in reality, I'm anxious over nothing at all. Nothing has happened yet in the present. These feelings are due to forward thinking. Sometimes, you might convince yourself you're going to feel bad before you even perform that action, visit that place, see that person or encounter that trigger. You may even start avoiding that "thing" because you think it'll make the anxiety go away or prevent it from getting worse. All you're doing is reinforcing how important it is. You're teaching your brain it's something to be scared of when in reality, it's not. You might find yourself pulling at strings, looking for an indication that the fear is valid. Perhaps you're hyperaware of your surroundings and look for "signs" around you, or listen in conversations with friends and family for something that signifies your anxious thoughts are real and true.

I've managed to convince myself that inhabiting my own apartment is destined to go wrong. There are a lot of unknowns associated with being in a new environment. I don't know how I'm going to feel or adapt. Change triggers my anxiety—change of scenery, lifestyle changes, or diet/exercise changes. Moving out of my childhood home is the ultimate test. I've lived in New York City my whole life. I only moved a mile away from my family. My boyfriend works a few blocks away. I know this neighborhood like the back of my hand. But somehow, this new life feels strange and unfamiliar.

When I feel "off" mentally, my brain reads it as being in danger, and I'll have a strong physical reaction. I get dizzy and have a hard time concentrating. It becomes difficult to follow conversations as I fall down a rabbit hole of rumination. Moving into my own space is lonelier than I expected. I'm having serious anxiety being alone, and I'm craving someone to keep me company.

I hate feeling codependent. It takes me back to my childhood: I had attachment issues as a kid. I would never leave my mom's side, and my growth into an adult was stunted as a result. I thought separating myself from her was for my own good, but I'll admit, I do miss her. The lack of activity in the apartment freaks me out. I'm my own source of entertainment. My mom isn't around pestering me to film TikToks. My dad isn't blasting football games on the television. It's just me, alone with my thoughts. I can't count how many naps I've taken over the past few days to pass the time.

Don't get me wrong: I have no regrets over my choice to move out. In fact, I was the one who prompted myself to take the leap. I blame the delay on being an only child. I dodged sleepaway camp. I lived at home throughout college. Staying with my parents was the norm. It was comfortable and familiar. Although living in New York City helped me gain independence, I knew I wouldn't feel like a real adult until I got out from under their roof. They still see me as their baby. There was no way they'd ever kick me out of the house. I had to start making mature decisions for the benefit of my future self. I needed to stop relying on my parents and start standing on my own two feet. I booked the apartment tours. I negotiated with brokers. I got my learner's permit and started taking driving lessons so I could take myself around. I put the work in because I knew that if I didn't, it would become increasingly harder to let go. I'm about to be a college graduate with a full-time job. It's time to start making my own choices.

Adulthood has approached so fast that I'm having trouble processing it. I blast Tate McRae's album loud enough to not hear my anxious thoughts. I work out so long, so hard, that the only growing pains I feel are in my legs. It feels like the world is spinning a web of stress I can't seem to untangle. How will I have enough money for three meals a day, seven days a week? What happens if I get locked out of my apartment? Or if I break a glass and nobody's there to help me clean up?

Adulting hits like a tsunami—it crashes over you when you least expect it. Like when I had my first panic attack weeks before my eighteenth birthday. Or when I lost my grandma. Adulting can simultaneously be exciting and scary. I think about how I met my boyfriend almost a year ago, and now I can't imagine my life without him. Or how an internship fulfilled my dream of writing for a newspaper.

That said, in the more difficult moments, it's hard to stay rational. Reason is often dismissed in the face of anxiety. So how do we stay grounded when everything around us is moving at light speed? In my case, I try to acknowledge the pros of having my own apartment: independence, freedom, and more me time. No more parents interrupting me or dog barking while I'm trying to write. I now have my own personal space, and I feel very fortunate. I'm trying to embrace the calm and find peace in the silence instead of being scared of it.

The answer to staying grounded is love: self-love, love for others, and gratitude for the role they have played in your growth. I take a second to appreciate my constants, both human and material. I hug my parents extra tight and tell them how much I love them. I add an extra twenty minutes onto my workout. I savor the last bite of nigiri from my favorite neighborhood sushi spot.

I'll also let you in on a little secret. When I'm feeling helpless, I listen to old voicemails of my grandma telling me she loves and misses me. It's a poignant reminder that no matter how life shakes you, love is never lost.

SELF-CARE CORNER:
THE LITTLE THINGS

Facing anxiety is fundamentally the mind's work. However, there are certain tools to help you along your recovery. The basics are most important; getting good sleep, staying fed and hydrating throughout the day keeps symptoms in check. Incorporating objects for anxiety relief can only further help. When I started doing exposure therapy, my therapist advised me to seek out something calming that would engage my five senses after the session. Here are some of my favorite finds that have supported me on my journey and may assist you, too.

- Purble: a stuffed animal with a rapid heartbeat. As you pet its head, the heartbeat slows, and yours along with it.

- CalmiGo: a device that guides you through breathing with lights and vibration cues.

- Rescue Pastilles: lozenges infused with flower essence for natural stress relief.

- Lavender essential oil: a relaxing scent proven to ease symptoms of anxiety. Rub two to three drops on your wrists or temples for optimal benefits.

- Peloton meditation: a collection of classes on the fitness app dedicated to relaxation and recentering. The Peloton library offers meditation classes focused on breathing, calming, sleep, and anxiety relief.

- Stress ball: a fidget toy used to "squeeze out" your stress and improve focus in the short term.

- Sour candy: intended to relieve anxiety and panic attacks by distracting the brain. You become focused on feeling rather than thinking when the strong sour flavor hits.

- A "calm" playlist: a collection of your favorite songs that puts you in a relaxing state of mind. My playlist includes Alec Benjamin, Olivia Rodrigo, Tate McRae, and Lewis Capaldi.

CHAPTER 11
REBOUND

I thought I knew better. I thought I made progress and had a greater understanding of my OCD than ever before. And then boom—a new intrusive thought hit. Just when I'd moved on from one battle, the next one struck. I thought I had the tools to handle it. I knew I shouldn't have confessed the intrusive thought. But putting my negative thoughts into the universe, no matter how it might affect others, seemed like the only way to alleviate guilt. Little did I know the guilt and anxiety would transfer onto the person I confessed to. And the feeling of guilt from deflecting is far worse, in my opinion.

Let me provide some context. I'm on a trip to Las Vegas right now, and while I sat in the sauna, I remembered something I said to a family member several months ago about a person close to me. I couldn't remember if I had actually said it the way I thought, but from what I recalled, it was mean. It made me feel like a bad person. I ruminated over the memory and wondered what the subject of my comments would think of me if they knew what I said.

I get mad at myself when it'ws been a long time since I confessed an OCD thought and suddenly, I get a strong urge. It usually happens on vacation. Like clockwork, my surroundings change, and my anxiety is rekindled. I'll look through photos or text messages to bring myself back to reality, but the reassurance-seeking becomes compulsive. I'm well aware of this pattern by now, but each time presents a new and seemingly impossible challenge to conquer.

I'm deliberately not revealing the content of the thought because, yes, it's private, but most importantly, it's irrelevant, intrusive and against what I truly believe. My impulse to confess the mean thought to the person I said it about months later was random. Its sudden recurrence, as well as the intense urge I had to confess, was proof to me that this was simply something my anxiety was latching onto—not actually something to worry about. If what I said all those months ago was an actual concern, I would think more about it instead of just wanting to blurt it out.

My therapist tells me that if I can't avoid confessing completely, I should try to wait as long as possible before doing so. The idea is that over time, the confession is delayed more and more until it doesn't need to be said at all. After what I considered a not-so-impressive few hours of keeping that memory to myself, I confessed it to the person that the intrusive thought was centered around. Confessing may temporarily relieve my guilt at the moment, but it's selfish. I'm not considering how my words will impact others before I say them.

It's as if I'm in survival mode, and I can't function unless my brain stops screaming with intrusive thoughts. It feels like I'm in danger if I don't speak up, when in reality, I'm perfectly safe. The brain is giving me a false alarm. Luckily, the person I confessed the intrusive thought to was close enough to me to understand that I was caught in an OCD cycle. Although they didn't have a strong reaction, they did seem annoyed and told me that confessing would not be of service for either of us. They encouraged me to shift my intention and observe my thoughts non-judgmentally instead of fighting them. I would acknowledge they are there, thank them for working to keep me safe, and choose not to further engage.

I'm told to be compassionate with myself if I lose to my OCD by confessing intrusive thoughts. Progress is not linear. The problem for me, though, is not practicing patience. I took three months off from running after finding out I had stress fractures—you'd think I'd have the patience of a saint. The problem is I worry that people won't be patient with me. As irrational as it may sound, my OCD convinces me that the people I love will leave. I fear I'll lose everyone I love most because they'll get sick of hearing my intrusive thoughts and start to believe they'll never subside. How am I supposed to believe I'll get better if nobody else does?

That itself is an intrusive thought. The people who love me and know about my OCD believe in me and promise they won't give up. I'm grateful but still skeptical. Even though I know my intrusive thoughts aren't real, I worry that deep down, others might think so. I fear they might be piecing the intrusive thoughts I've confessed together to try to form some "truth." In reality, although my intrusive thoughts may be similar in content, each one stands alone, and never, ever, do they hold truth.

I'll be honest. In moments of high anxiety, I hate myself. I hate that I can't "heal" fast enough. I hate that I keep making the same mistakes. I hate that my loved ones have to keep watching it happen. I have a hard time believing someone can love me while I'm flawed.

A particular memory comes to mind. I lost a friend because of my anxiety. When I was first experiencing panic attacks in 2020, she stayed at my house for my birthday weekend. She traveled all the way from Los Angeles to celebrate with me. I wanted to be present for her. I wanted to be the upbeat, extroverted friend she knew and loved. But I just couldn't. All I wanted to do was curl up on the couch and stare at my phone to distract myself from what was going on in my mind. I tried to explain what was happening, but she didn't seem to understand. Anxiety is unique to the individual, so it was hard to put what I was feeling into words she could grasp.

She suggested activities that she was interested in (arts and crafts, scrapbooking, baking) and didn't listen to me or my needs. The only things making me feel better were social media and fitness. She didn't want to engage in those, so I spent most of my time alone. All I wanted was for her to be there for me, to ask how I was feeling and what she could do to help. Instead, I had to be there for myself.

Turns out, that friend resented me for not spending enough time with her. She did not show me grace in the face of my struggles. In fact, she ghosted me, and when she picked up the phone months later, she said she could no longer be the friend I wanted her to be. I felt like my anxiety sent her running. I pictured a sign taped to my back: "Mentally ill. Do not engage." Some people don't know how to handle anxiety in themselves or others, which is what I believe pushed her away. Perhaps she was going through something, and hearing about my anxiety was too much for her to handle. It's tough to pinpoint exactly what tore us apart, but I do know that a real friend would tell you why they're walking away.

It feels like everybody and nobody understands what I'm going through. The world preaches "mental health matters," yet why do I feel so alone sometimes? I often find myself wondering what everyone is thinking. Do they hate me as much as I hate myself when I'm having an anxious episode? Are they as scared as I am?

I now understand that the most valuable friends are the ones who are there for you at your worst and don't flee when the going gets tough. My best friend sat on my bed with me for hours as I sobbed into her shoulder in 2020. My other friend no longer lives a few blocks away, but she's always there to pick up the phone when I need to rant. There are good people out there. You just have to be patient. It's frustrating that in 2024, we still have to explain what it means to have OCD. Luckily, my loved ones make an effort to learn, and I'm patient with them as they try to understand my disorder. It creates the opportunity for deep conservations and emotionally rich relationships.

As I previously mentioned, I'm in Vegas right now. I've been writing this in between excursions and activities: while waiting for a Styx concert to start, foam rolling at the gym, and sitting at the casino. After days of playing slots with no luck, I just cashed out $300. It looks like betting on myself is easier than I thought.

SELF-CARE CORNER:

NORMALIZE MAKING MISTAKES

Conquering anxiety and OCD is not as simple as just telling yourself to "stop." No matter how hard you try to resist compulsions, you will most likely disappoint yourself. You will fail. But you will fail forward.

A week may go by when you're doing well: your OCD and anxiety symptoms are in check. The frustrating thing about anxiety, though, is that you never know when it's going to strike, and when it does, you might feel unprepared. You might not handle it as well as you did the last time it came up. Anxiety is not a straight, upward slope. It fluctuates. Everyone has good days and bad days. A bad day doesn't mean you're losing progress.

The more mistakes become normalized in your mind, the easier they'll be to tackle. With disorders as tricky as OCD and GAD, it's unrealistic to set high standards for recovery right away. Show yourself grace in the face of your slip-ups. Give yourself time, patience, and a pat on the back for putting in effort, especially when life gets heavy.

CHAPTER 12
LONELY

OCD is lonely. I can't begin to express the intense feelings of isolation when my anxiety is brewing. I feel depersonalized as I sit here on my sofa. I see others smiling outside my window and wonder how their minds are so clear, so happy. Why does it feel like I'm the only struggling?

No matter how much I want to ask for help, when I do, I often feel misunderstood. I text my therapist first in SOS moments. Talking through my mental health with a medical professional brings perspective to my life. Unlike chats with a friend, a therapist is solely intended to help you by using their education and expertise. My therapist doesn't tell me what to do or how to think. She asks questions and prompts me to look deep within myself to find my own answers. However, at times, therapy is frustrating. I wish my therapist could just tell me how to resolve my anxiety and feel better. I do most of the talking during our appointments when I really want to learn from her. I want our sessions to be less emotional, more educational—but that's not her strategy. The awkward silences when she wants me to continue the conversation are agonizing. Outside of our sessions, when I text to ask for help, her response is: "That's frustrating. Would you like to schedule a call?"

Therapy varies from person to person, and your relationship with therapy may transform over time. It feels different for me than it did in 2020. In the beginning, my sessions sustained me. My therapist was the only one who really knew about my anxiety, so I looked forward to talking to her. I was also doing exposure therapy at the time, which she was monitoring. Now that I'm more open about my anxiety with friends and family, therapy doesn't serve the same purpose. Lately, it's been more of a slow burn. Although the self-reflection in my sessions strengthens my mental health over time, in the moment, it doesn't alleviate my anxiety. My therapist taught me the basics of OCD, but I want to continue learning. She gives me the same advice over and over again: "Engage your five senses to ground yourself, move your body, and spend time with loved ones."

So I turn to my mom, which I wind up regretting. It's not her fault: it's her job as a mother to try to problem-solve. Nobody wants to admit their daughter is struggling. As much as she tries to relate ("I have anxiety, too!"), she does not understand because she does not experience OCD like I do. The way she responds to my anxiety flare-ups is by asking about the specific content of my intrusive thoughts, which is never productive. If I confess the thoughts to her, she tries to disprove them or renders them silly—also unproductive. They're not silly to me. They're deeply disturbing and upsetting. "They're garbage thoughts," she'll say to me, even though I'm aware. I know she means well in reassuring me, but it feels like she's saying what she thinks she's supposed to say rather than listening to how I feel. I don't think she knows what to say, so she relays metaphors that her own therapist told her. I can't tell you how many times she's referred to my anxiety as a false fire alarm. The analogies don't usually resonate. It's moments like these when I feel particularly lonely. It seems that as soon as I get the courage to reach out for help, it backfires, and I feel more misunderstood. I just assume it's the universe's plan. Maybe the lack of help is a sign that no help was ever needed, because everything is already fine.

My dad used to be my number one confidant because he's very non-alarmist. I could tell him the most disturbing intrusive thought and he'd shrug it off. "I get it," he'd tell me. "You have that track always running around your brain. It's happened to me before, too." I can't confide in him, though. Everything I say I know will be relayed to my mom. Nothing ever remains between us. As much as I love him, he's not good at keeping secrets. Equally frustrating: if I go a month without talking to him about my anxiety, he automatically assumes it's "gone." He thinks that me not talking about it means I'm "all better." He doesn't consider that maybe I just don't want to talk about it. I'm at peace with the fact that even though my parents are always there for support, they will never fully understand how I'm feeling. So I typically just stay silent.

Then there's my boyfriend, who is willing to protect me at all costs. He's the one person who has ever truly understood my anxiety. He's smart. He knows me well. He can sense the second I'm in an anxious mindset as I start picking at my knuckles. "Everything will be okay," he tells me, kissing my fingers one by one. If I try to pretend I'm fine, he immediately senses I'm off and encourages me to confront my emotions. He has sat with me through several panic attacks and brought me back to the present. He grounds me. He helps pick up the pieces when I don't have the strength to. He loves me for both my scars and my sunshine.

Here's the kicker: It hurts. Loving him is beautiful, but it hurts me that I have to show him my greatest weakness and insecurity. It hurts that he has to hold me while

I fall apart in his arms. It hurts that the empath he is has to feel every tear, every anxious pang as I do. My first true love, my soulmate, has to live with my anxiety if he wants to spend his life with me. I feel guilty. It's unfair to him. Sometimes, I push away panic attacks and stifle tears so he doesn't think there's something wrong with me. I hold back because I don't want to scare him. But I try to remind myself that anxiety is nothing to be ashamed of, nor is it contagious. I don't have to feel sorry for laying my feelings on the line or worry about transferring them to him. Talking about mental health is a big help. Holding back your emotions doesn't make you any stronger.

I'm still actively trying to accept my anxiety. I believe it's my life's journey. This is the challenge G-d has given me. I am so grateful for His blessings. He gave me legs that run marathons, hands that write novels, and the capacity to love others with all my heart. But I'm far from perfect. Nobody can have it all.

As much as I put on a show on social media, the girl behind the upbeat TikTok unboxings struggles sometimes. She loves her career, but she doesn't love the anxiety that comes with it. She is grateful, but her days can also be dark and gloomy. She loves to talk, but sometimes the fear of saying too much suffocates her. People expect me to be happy all the time just because of the opportunities I've been given. Of course I'm grateful, but that's a lot of pressure to put on one girl. Let's normalize not being okay all the time. Nobody is superhuman. It's about balance. Joy and anxiety can coexist. The longer I stand in that truth, the easier it gets.

Everyone gets intrusive thoughts. Tell me you haven't wondered what would happen if a car hit you as you crossed the street, or if your finger got too close to the flame when cooking. But not everyone feels the intense urge to confess these thoughts, as if something bad will happen if they don't. I fear self-sabotage by accepting intrusive thoughts as truth. I worry that OCD will succeed in convincing me that the thoughts are real and prevent me from achieving lasting happiness. I don't ever want to give into the thoughts, but the noisier they are, the more daunting they feel. Wishing things were better and worrying about my thoughts is a major time and energy suck. I spend so much time stuck on intrusive thoughts, sitting still with my eyes closed in rumination. It's challenging to stay present when my brain is running a million miles a minute.

OCD craves certainty. It'll ask, "how do you know that intrusive thought isn't what you actually believe?" Or "why don't we logic through this to double-check that you're sure?" It's nicknamed "the doubting disorder" for a reason. The truth is that your gut already knows the answer. You know yourself and your core values better than anyone. You are not responsible for your intrusive thoughts.

Instead of panicking, I'm learning to practice response prevention. That includes not always checking in on my feelings or ruminating over my obsessions. Rather than trying to answer the illogical questions OCD raises, I shrug them off with "maybe." I read on Instagram that falling in love with "maybe" is one of the best things you can do for your anxiety. When OCD poses a question, you answer with "maybe," and the outcome doesn't seem as alarming. For example: maybe you were a little annoying at that party. Maybe that itchy throat really does mean you're sick. But probably not. The word "maybe" is casual enough to help you shrug off your fears.

THERAPIST'S COUCH:
RESPONSE PREVENTION

According to Nathan Peterson, OCD Therapist and Licensed Clinical Social Worker

Response prevention is deliberately choosing not to engage with your compulsions. It involves responding to intrusive thoughts with phrases like, "maybe" or "maybe not" when OCD threatens disaster. This technique sends signals back to the brain that say, "I know you're telling me I'm in danger right now, but let me test this out to see if you're wrong."

OCD wants you to know for sure if your fear is accurate or not, so it doesn't like when you agree with its unfounded threats. For example, if OCD says, "You're going to get sick," and you respond, "I sure hope so. How about I touch that subway pole and deliberately forget to wash my hands this time?" Resisting and delaying compulsions sends signals to the brain that teach you you're not actually in danger. Facing your fears may feel uncomfortable in the moment, but practicing response prevention will gradually teach your brain that there is no need to perform the compulsion.

I know my intrusive thoughts are OCD because of the OCD behaviors I exhibit outside of them. I often get caught in a loop of physical compulsions. They're not the same ones as 2022, but I have started recognizing patterns in my OCD over time. Although the Notes app essays have come to a close, I instead obsess over emails, endlessly scrolling through the trash to ensure I didn't delete anything important. I double-check if photos are sorted into the correct folders in my camera roll. When I look at an email or photo and feel like I'm ready to delete it, I get stuck. The information I'm reading never feels like it fully registers—like a ball hitting the wall that doesn't penetrate.

Recognizing patterns brings me peace. When I have a strong urge to confess an intrusive thought, I think back to years prior, when I had a similar inclination to reveal a different thought. In both instances, I was burdened by thoughts I don't believe. Coming to this realization attaches less guilt to the OCD. It helps me accept that these habits are simply part of a disorder. They mean nothing about who you are.

Compulsions tend to be worse on days when I'm bored and have "nothing better to do" (there's always a way to be productive). Sometimes, I stay up late double-checking to the point where my head hurts from eye strain. I wait until my mind feels "just right" and I feel positive that I edited every piece of footage I filmed for TikTok that day—but can you ever be really sure? You must settle for "maybe." What you're "missing" in that email or camera role is hypothetical and unlikely. But what you're gaining is much more valuable—time, and even sleep.

Sometimes, to separate from the compulsion, I'll often set an ultimatum: "If you stop looking at your camera roll for the rest of the day, you'll have good luck." Or "if you keep scrolling through your emails, you're going to have bad luck." I'll count down from three and stop performing the compulsion. Although it temporarily works, it's tricky because falling back on superstitions becomes a compulsion in itself. This type of wishful thinking is not productive. There is no correlation between photos or emails and luck. Lying to myself in saying that there is just adds pressure to not slip up, and it intensifies feelings of shame when I fail.

I've learned how to fake being okay—it's a talent, really. People assume I'm just obsessed with my phone when really, I spend hours checking and double-checking things that are unnecessary. They'll tell me I'm "so organized," but they have no idea how time spent organizing drains my energy.

I prioritize taking care of myself when my OCD spikes. Self-care is more than just a warm shower and a cup of hot cocoa. It involves embracing your passions and personal needs. To me, taking care of myself means going on a long run. It includes making time to sit at my computer and write, even when my day is packed with appointments. The grass is greener where you water it. Sitting back and waiting for things to get better won't work. The more you dedicate yourself to furthering your peace and happiness, the more progress you'll make in bettering your mental health. I try to remind myself that living with a mental health disorder doesn't mean good days are gone.

SELF-CARE CORNER:

ASK YOURSELF QUESTIONS

Getting too deeply immersed in your anxiety isn't always the best idea. However, confronting yourself with basic questions (ones that have "yes/no" or one-word answers) actually simplifies what's going on inside your brain. If your answer to a question is "no," it shows you that the thought is probably not worth your energy. Meeting your mind with a question can help untangle things and calm you down. Think about it: intrusive thoughts are swirling, and you stop to ask yourself if you can be doing something better with your time. It puts your anxiety in perspective and moves you forward. Having a set of questions ready when you find yourself ruminating can bring you back to reality. Try keeping some (or all) of the below in your toolkit.

- Is this a helpful thought?
- Does this thought define who I am?
- Does this thought resonate with me?
- Who am I independent of this thought?
- Do I need to think about this right now?

- Can I be doing something more productive?
- Is this thought 100 percent true?
- How does this thought make me feel?
- Does this thought add value to my day?
- Is this thought taking me away from the present moment?
- Would I feel better if I stopped thinking about this?
- Is this worth spending time worrying about?

in reality, I was just offering to spotlight her small business. She posted screenshots of our messages and called me a "scammer" and "fraud." This false narrative about me went viral on TikTok, garnering millions of views. I received thousands of comments on my videos shaming me, as well as negative direct messages on Instagram. Many of those messages were, indeed, death threats.

A little girl sent me about fifty DMs with the same word written over and over again: "die." Another profile with a bio reading "mom of two beautiful baby girls" said that the world would be better off without me. Here I was, coping with intrusive thoughts about suicide, and people were "validating" the anxiety by telling me to die. The words swirling in my head made their way onto strangers' phones, and I assumed that gave my intrusive thoughts a sense of truth. Back then, I couldn't zoom out to acknowledge just how awful it was that a child and mother were sending these messages. I was so deep in the anxiety, all I focused on was existing from day to day.

My therapist helped me cope with the messages through desensitization. The DMs were little text bubbles; when flipped on their side and strung together, they almost looked like a caterpillar. She colored the bubbles in green and drew on a head to reinforce the comparison. The caterpillar screenshot remains on my desktop to this day in case I need a reminder that strangers' hateful words are meaningless. Yes, the strategy was silly, but it made me smile. It showed me that at the end of the day, texts are texts, and they're only what you make of them. Plus, the people who wrote them don't even know me. These are complete strangers who have never met me and probably never will. Their opinions don't matter.

After about three weeks of being "canceled," the internet moved on to their next victim. I was relieved, but I was left with a mess to clean up mentally. The worst type of hate is self-hate—you're your own worst enemy. When the attacks finally calmed down, I was left with was a diminished sense of self-worth. In these moments, I have to get in touch with my central confidence. It took me years to develop my self-confidence—high school bullies and backstabbing ballerinas at dance class gave me a tough skin. I know it's there. It's just more difficult to channel when the words around me are so hostile and loud.

To come back to center, I direct my attention to activities I love most—writing, running, biking. I show myself how strong I am and make a conscious effort to boost my endorphins. You may feel insecure when someone is hating on you. It's a normal, logical reaction, but it's not a good idea to do so for too long. You have no control over the other person, but you do have control over yourself and how you handle the rest of your day. I find it's best to handle the bully as calmly and strategically as possible, and if they still won't let up, it's not worth wasting any more of your energy. I give myself an hour or two to do damage control, and if alleviating the situation isn't feasible, I keep it where it is. I don't reach too far because I know that if I do, I'll break.

Getting hated on is common, but that doesn't make it any more acceptable. You never know what someone is going through and how your words might affect them. The death threats I received brought my already intense anxiety to a whole new level. No stranger deserved the power to make me feel the way I did. A lot of the time, the problem isn't even about you. Hurt people hurt people. Try to shift your perspective and realize that every verbal attack thrown your way makes you stronger. Yes, the words sting, but they leave behind battle scars. The situations we struggle over and endure supercharge us so that next time, the hate may not cut as deep. The anxiety may not emerge as vigorously. You may shrug instead of sob. You may laugh instead of linger over messages. You will recognize that these people may have tried to hurt you, but your sense of self was never really lost.

SELF-CARE CORNER:

DEALING WITH BULLIES

I've been bullied since I was in elementary school. It's exhausting, really. You'd think at this point, I'd finally catch a break. I've learned that the more I continue to stay independent and driven, the more of a target I become. People love to pick on those who are successful.

Being bullied sucks. I spent my entire four years of high school hiding in the library so I didn't have to confront any of my peers who mocked me and my writing career. I wound up quitting dance after finding out that my "best friends" had a group chat where they trashed me behind my back. Being prone to anxiety only makes the hate sting more, as you ruminate over whether the bully's words hold meaning. Luckily, the amount of hate I've gotten over the years has trained me to conquer bullies well when they arise. Here are some of my tips for taking them on.

1. Never match their level of hostility. Getting defensive only makes matters worse, especially if they're already angry. Approach the situation with a sense of calm and a willingness to talk things out.

2. Don't take anything too personally. Bullies almost always have something else going on in their lives that make them insecure and eager to attack others.

3. Don't say anything your future self wouldn't be proud of. Emotions run high when hateful words are spewed at you, but try your best to remain level-headed and respectful.

4. Step away from the situation. Taking space from the site of the hate can bring you perspective and help recenter you.

5. Phone a friend. Sometimes, you just need to rant. Call and tell them what's going through your head. They may even offer some great advice.

6. Focus on rebuilding your confidence. When a bully knocks you down, the best thing to do is reunite with your passion. Take on an activity that makes you happy and benefits your future self.

7. Be patient and remember that things will get better. Bullies may have stamina, but they won't target you forever. Take a deep breath and calmly wait for the storm to pass.

CHAPTER 14
CHAOTIC

Life used to move slowly with my anxiety. The days felt long and tedious—I would count the hours until night-time so I could unwind. Lately, life is moving quickly, and that hasn't made it any easier to handle.

The opportunity to plan international trips recently arose—Japan, Costa Rica, Australia. I'm grateful that I have the ability to travel, but the unknown makes me anxious. I've never traveled out of the country without my family. Embarrassingly, I've never even booked my own flight. How am I supposed to figure out an entire itinerary? Will finances be an issue? I'm in a weird in-be-tween state right now career-wise. It feels like the world is my oyster, yet I can't seem to land a full-time journalism job. With my college graduation soon approaching, the lack of security is scary. Looking ahead to a year full of potential trips, a lot worries me. I'm nervous that I'll plan a vacation, and all of a sudden, I'll secure a job and have to cancel at the last minute. There's no way I'm taking a trip during my first week of work.

On top of that, there's my generalized travel anxiety. Going to a new state in the U.S. throws me for a loop, but there's a sense of familiarity in my own country. Places I've been before are not a problem. Traveling hours outside of North America makes me feel like I'm stepping outside of myself and into a new world, a new civilization. On one hand, it's exciting. I get to learn about people, places, and things I've never seen before and see life through a different lens. But being in a new place makes me feel out of control. I don't know what the people are going to be like. I don't know how the food is going to taste. It's not my ordinary routine. As my mom likes to say, I'm not someone who likes my cheese moved—not down the street, not to a new state, and certainly not thousands of miles away.

I hold onto the things in my life that are familiar. I generally eat the same foods every week (chicken salad is a must). I go through the same workout rotation (running, cycling and lifting). I watch at least thirty minutes of TV before bed. A sense of routine keeps me sane. If one small area of my life is adjusted (for example, incorporating a new snack during the day), my anxiety is easily triggered.

It's frustrating. Why can't I just be more open to change? Even a change as positive as visiting a new country stresses me out. It challenges my rules and rituals and temporarily replaces them. I think back to a moment on a recent cruise I went on to the Bahamas. The stars above the ship were beautiful. My boyfriend led me in a dance around the top deck with nobody around. Yet I wasn't able to fully soak in and enjoy the moment. The change in scenery triggered me, and I could only focus on how anxious I was feeling.

Trying to explain this to friends and loved ones seems impossible. "What's stressful about a beautiful tropical vacation?" they say. "This shouldn't be anxiety-inducing." Telling me I "should" or "shouldn't" feel a certain way is not a productive way to move forward. I can't always control my anxiety. I didn't ask for it to be there.

I'll spend hours expressing why trips scare me. I typically grow emotional. It's scary to admit that my apprehension about vacation isn't just the money or worries about missing work. It's my mental health. I feel guilty using it as an excuse, but the reality is that it affects several areas of my life, whether I want it to or not.

That doesn't mean I won't ever go on trips. It doesn't mean I'll hold back from international travel and avoid leaving New York at all costs. It just means that I'm not as quick to book airline tickets as others might be. It means that I may have some silent moments on the trip because I'm alone in my thoughts and struggling. It's sad and it sucks.

I recently started planning a trip to Australia with some friends. It was very stressful at first. This is a place I've never been before, that I'm entirely unfamiliar with. I knew I'd be flying blind. I planned my trip slower than everybody else. Instead of jumping into buying plane tickets the same day the trip was proposed, I wanted to wait. Rather than shopping for an Airbnb, I decided that I wanted my own space.

I actually wound up surprising myself. I became so invested in the trip that I planned a group spa day for everyone. Nobody else seemed to be researching activities as much as I was. I was proud of how I threw myself into the vacation, even when it made me uncomfortable.

Ultimately, my friends decided not to do a group trip to Australia. There was too much dissension. It felt like it was my fault. I was humiliated. I was the only one putting effort into research for Australia. I was planning activities for the entire group to enjoy. It seemed like I was punished for being cautious about booking. I have a book to write, four social media pages to run, and a race to train for. I needed to iron out details before dropping hundreds of dollars on a plane ticket.

Stressors aside, I was still all-in on Australia. I ignored my anxiety and dove in head first. Nobody cared or appreciated it. In their eyes, the baby of the group was holding everyone back from confirming transportation and housing, and they worried I would only become a further hindrance.

I felt defenseless. Nobody seemed to care about my career situation; they all had no problem taking vacation time off work. Plus, there was no way I would admit to them that I was working through travel anxiety. I was going out of my way to make this trip happen when internally, I was freaking out. I assumed if I was honest with them, they would have just seen my anxiety as an excuse. They would never understand.

I try to practice patience with myself, because that's the only way others are going to be patient with me. I'm still working on my travel anxiety. Each trip I agree to go on is a step in the right direction. I'm even thinking about flying to Tokyo next year with my boyfriend. When it comes to future travels, I trust that the people who love me will be patient with me. I attempt to stay as grounded as possible in explaining my mental health situation, even though it's a huge challenge. Oftentimes, I'm embarrassed. Telling people I can't commit to vacations right away due to anxiety makes me feel ashamed. I trust that my loved ones will help me through trips and be privy to the fact that I'm highly sensitive to change. Those who don't make an effort to understand or support how my brain is wired aren't people I'd want to travel with anyway.

Traveling in groups is popular, especially as you enter your twenties. Sure, group trips can be fun. What I'm learning is that just because you're jetting off with a crew doesn't mean you have to sacrifice who you are. I am a career-driven individual who can't just pick up and leave for a week at the drop of a hat. I am also an anxious individual who can't agree to planning a major vacation without seriously thinking things through. You should never apologize for who you are.

SELF-CARE CORNER:
RELAXATION

Anxiety can make it seem like everything and everyone is against you. Intrusive thoughts are raging, your surroundings are spinning, and you can't manage to stay present. In these moments, make a deliberate choice to calm yourself down. Doing so can be difficult, especially if you're mid-panic. But having relaxing objects close by in a situation when you know you might be triggered can help. Try smelling essential oils or playing with fidget toys to center your mind. If you're at home, turn on your favorite television show or follow an online meditation.

There are dozens of stress-relief objects on the market to guide you: therapy putty, plushies, sensory rings, cooling face masks, and more. But all it really takes to relax is you and your breath. It's important to learn how to calm yourself down in case those objects are out of reach. If you're out in public and anxiety strikes, step away for a moment and close your eyes. Listen to your breaths, and count them until you feel your heart rate slow down. Force yourself to breathe, even when it feels hard or you don't want to. Once you assert that power over yourself, you'll realize that you have more control over your reaction to anxiety than you thought.

CHAPTER 15
CHANGED

As much as memories from 2020 still sting, a lot of what occurred seems distant. All I hoped for back then was to move forward, to step into a new skin where anxiety did not burden me every day. Yes, I still struggle, but the pain doesn't cut as deeply as it used to. Now, I'm about to graduate college, and I feel like a different person. This can't be that same girl who sat trembling in her bed, scared of hurting herself just four years ago. Where did that part of myself go? It couldn't have just disappeared.

I wonder if there are memories locked away that I'm simply too scared to face. I read old journals and quickly move on for fear of reverting to a similar mindset. Do we give up the person we once were to embrace the person we are now? Or will that person always be inside? You will always shed a part of who you are to become who you're destined to be. Your core values tend to stay stationary. But you have to give up parts of yourself in order to grow—it's crucial. Otherwise, you will remain stuck.

Memories are never really gone—they're always accessible. It's just a matter of opening your mind and allowing yourself to feel them. I don't buy the "I can't remember" excuse. Memories may be in the past, but they will always be a part of your story. The person I was in 2020 is not who I am anymore. But if I allow my mind to wander back to that place, I can access those memories.

If I close my eyes, I can feel her: the anxious teenager scared of turning eighteen because she doesn't know what the world has to offer, or what she has to offer the world. I don't listen to her often because those feelings are too tough to confront. As much as I've grown, that anxious teenager will always be a part of my memory. She comes to visit, whether I like it or not—like when I moved into a new apartment, or when I realized I was falling in love.

I prefer to keep memories attached to my anxious episodes locked away. I don't remember every detail, nor do I want to. I avoid people and places related to moments when I was at my worst so that I don't get triggered. It's unproductive if I want to desensitize myself over time, but definitely the easier route. Ironically, with other smaller, more insignificant life events, I find myself memory hoarding. The fact that I can't remember every detail of my past makes me anxious and uneasy. It's actually a symptom of OCD.

Memory hoarding is just another compulsion. I feel like I need to capture every moment perfectly in case the memory needs to be recalled in the future. Oftentimes, when I obsess over a memory, it's to ensure I didn't make a mistake and say or do anything wrong. Other times, it's to confirm a positive memory is fully stored away so I can call upon it when needed. The ritual can become overwhelming. I replay a moment over and over again in my mind to see if I remember. I scroll through photos or text messages for reassurance. But even when I seemingly get that reassurance, somehow, my brain is unsatisfied.

Looking back, I feel like writing *My Real-Life Rom-Com* may have been a form of memory hoarding. As much as processing past relationships on the page was therapeutic, I feel like I obsessed over capturing every detail of my past. I tried to remember what exactly a guy said to me that made me feel special, or what he did that broke my heart. I wanted to store details because I worried I would never feel what it was like to love again. I didn't want to forget—so I wrote everything down. I assumed that even if I never found my person, at least I could relive the exciting encounters I had through the pages of my memoir.

Sometimes, I became so overly obsessed with collecting details, I would take notes in the middle of dates. When I went to the bathroom, I would jot down a few words and actions that resonated so they wouldn't be lost. Especially if I was having a good time, I wanted to bottle the feeling and save it for later.

What I've learned is that memories aren't supposed to be remembered perfectly. Life is meant to be enjoyed in the moment. Forgetting things is normal—it doesn't mean you're less worthy of living a fulfilling life, nor does it mean you can't hold onto memories. They arise at random times for me—like in a dream, or in the middle of the shower.

I have a hard time learning to let go of the fact that not everything can be remembered. However, I use it as inspiration to live in the moment more. The more I pay attention to what's going on in front of me, the more of a chance I have to retain the information. If I don't focus on what's being said to me in the present, how can I ever recall it in the future? Oftentimes, compulsively writing down details takes me out of the moment. I'd much rather risk not remembering something than abandon the present.

In the case of 2020, living in the present was tough. But I persevered, and honestly, it was for the better. Owning my emotions when they were at their strongest helped me come to terms with my OCD in a way that I probably should have a long time ago. Instead of ignoring the issue, I faced it head on. Those memories are far removed, but in the moment, they were very real. The fact that I shed a skin doesn't mean I'm abandoning the place where I once was. It means I've grown. My anxiety has matured. I have matured—and that's something I'm proud of.

I'm not confessing my intrusive thoughts as much. I'm not crying as often. But I still feel stuck. It feels like I'm waiting for someone to wave a magic wand and grant me complete peace of mind. Every morning, I open my eyes to find that there's no Fairy Godmother before me— just the same sticky, anxious feeling.

At this point, I know I'm going to be publishing these journal entries. I feel guilty that I'm not "cured," but I'm still championing mental health. I'm preaching about how to help yourself while I'm still broken. I often wonder, why speak out if I'm still working through my anxiety?

I felt like something was missing as I wrote this book. It seemed like something was left unsaid, a piece missing in this crazy puzzle that is presenting my mental health to the world. I think I found it: all this excitement over publishing another book has made me a bit restless. I'll admit it—I'm terrified. I've been honest about my struggles over the past few years, but I haven't talked much about what it's like to be putting the inner workings of your brain on blast.

I think of it like a math equation: me revealing my issues equals you hopefully speaking out to friends or family about what you're going through. No risk, no reward. It's not easy. I'm exposing myself. Letting people into my diary leaves me more raw, more vulnerable. I'll be easily susceptible to getting hurt. People's words will sting harder and faster. Emotions will run deeper. Do I really want to open the flood gates?

I'd like to say that people's words won't affect me, but I wonder what it will be like facing criticism from the crowd. Who am I to be giving advice when I'm not a doctor? I question if speaking up while I'm still struggling is premature.

But isn't that what being a champion is? Breaking down the walls? Making your voice heard even when anxiety is closing in on you? I'm not a therapist or psychologist, which often makes me feel like an imposter in the mental health space. But the difference between me and doctors is that I'm not just teaching the statistics—I am the statistic. I wish there were more people my age speaking out about their struggles with mental health and OCD. There's a void, and the silence is loud. I've always written my way out of pain—heartbreak, grief and now anxiety. Even though I'm scared, I want to do this. I think it's what I was destined to do. It feels like my calling.

When I was first experiencing panic attacks at the start of the pandemic, I refused to write about how I was feeling. My fingers were frozen. It was more than writer's block. It wasn't that there was a lack of inspiration. I was scared that if I wrote, the words on the page would reveal some truth about me that I didn't want to face. Admitting my mental health struggles on paper made them seem more real. I wasn't ready to admit I had a problem.

I told myself I would wait until I was "feeling better" before I wrote. I wanted to figure myself out and find my purpose first. I agonized over what that purpose was. I had just turned eighteen and the adult world ahead of me was intimidating. There were so many paths to choose from and questions to address. How would I find career success as a writer? Where would I meet my potential partner? Are my parents and I not going to be close anymore? Everything seemed unknown and daunting. Amid all the noise inside my head, one voice shot through: "What is this all for?"

Little did I know, my purpose was standing in front of me all along. The very thing I was avoiding at that time was what holds the most value in my life. My purpose is to write. My purpose is to stand in my truth and help others feel comfortable standing in theirs. Recognizing your purpose and stepping into it is terrifying. That's why writing this book has been so difficult for me. But I feel a sense of responsibility to represent my generation. This is what I have to do.

I've been struggling for years, but I've also accomplished a lot while I've been struggling. I ran a marathon. I published a book. I'm still here and succeeding. My brain might be screaming, but I still sustain myself. I keep fighting for myself. And I'm optimistic about the future.

I'm aware that your purpose changes over time. Eight-year-old Carrie was obsessed with cupcakes. Sixteen-year-old Carrie spearheaded her own fashion blog. Standing here at twenty-two, I'm as confident as ever that I want to be a journalist. The difference is that my career choice is now infused with a greater universal intention. I love reporting as much as I did when I was a teenager, if not more. But I also know that part of the reason I was placed on this Earth was to speak out about mental health. I don't have it all figured out yet. Nobody is supposed to have everything figured out. Part of being human is growing and changing and getting closer to becoming the person you're destined to be. Some risks may be involved (case in point: exposing your diary to millions of people worldwide), but harnessing your purpose is exciting. It's exhilarating. It makes life worth living.

SELF-CARE CORNER:

FORGIVE YOURSELF

Sometimes, I feel like a bad person for having intrusive thoughts. I tend to prescribe meaning to a thought if it's recurring. I tell myself, "If I'm thinking this terrible thought all the time, it's going to happen" or "it must be true." You are not responsible for the intrusive thoughts that enter your mind. They do not mean anything, and they most certainly do not define who you are.

But when they're so vivid and specific, you may forget they're an anxiety symptom. You can become so lost in a thought that you begin to convince yourself it's real. You can forget to separate thought from emotion and let the content consume you. By disengaging from the thought and merely letting it pass, you can teach the brain it's nothing to worry about.

However, recovery is more than just response prevention. The goal is to feel secure enough in yourself and your OCD that you practice self-compassion. Forgive yourself for your intrusive thoughts—no matter how dark, disturbing, sexual, immoral, or strange they are. You need to love yourself even, and especially, when you're feeling your worst. This involves being kind to yourself if you fail to resist a compulsion. It means not blaming yourself for the intrusive thoughts that arise.

Let go of the negative emotions attached to the disorder: guilt, anger, fear, disgust. When those feelings arise, give a competing response. Instead of wallowing in sadness, name three things you're grateful for. Rather than being frustrated, find peace through meditation. When you adopt a mindset of forgiveness and acceptance, you bring yourself closer to emotional healing. You begin to embrace that OCD and anxiety are not something you can change. You've conquered a lot more than the average person, but your battles callous you for life.

CHAPTER 16

PROGRESS

What now? It's the question I ask myself after every anxiety attack. When the symptoms subside and I come back down to Earth, I have a hard time determining where to turn. I tell myself to be productive. I force my feet into my running shoes. I place my hands on my computer keyboard and make myself write. I pick up the phone and call my mom and dad. Although I feel alone post-anxiety attack, I'm fortunate to have a lot of options for how to bring myself home.

Sometimes, I find myself praying. Not often—only when it matters, when I feel the most helpless and numb. Nobody knows I pray. I'm not super religious. I never have been. But when my light is stripped from me, I find myself naturally gravitating toward my roots, and it all starts with G-d. I'll ask for guidance. I'll pray. I'll plead. I'll pray some more. I'll cry quite a bit. But when I pray, something greater takes over. Sadness becomes serenity. Pain becomes perseverance. Hatred becomes hope. What once felt impossible now feels more manageable.

It's not a miracle by any means. I don't see prayer as some magic potion that suddenly obliterates anxiety. But it does help center me. It reminds me that although anxiety may feel hopeless at times, it's all a part of G-d's plan. It shows me that even when you feel alone, there will always be love—love from your parents, from a significant other, from friends, from whatever higher power you believe in. When anxiety strikes, the best way to fight it is with love.

I've noticed that in my current romantic relationship, talking about my anxiety is not met with fear or criticism. It's a safe space. I feel comfortable sharing a part of me that I'm not so proud of, and my partner embraces it with open arms. I feel very lucky to have found someone who encourages me to own my emotions and anxiety rather than push them down.

The first time I had an anxiety attack in front of my boyfriend, I was terrified. What if he thought I was crazy? What if I was too broken to love? I figured that if I was never enough for anyone before, there was no way I would ever be enough for him. My self-confidence had come a long way over the past few years, but my instinct at the prospect of losing this great love over my anxiety was to hide. I kept my breaths short and quiet. I ensured that my eyes stayed open extra wide because I knew the second I blinked, the tears would pour. Holding in my emotions hurt. I felt a mix of guilt, shame, fear, and sadness rising to the surface, ready to explode. I was so used to keeping it all to myself. I figured sharing would only further ignite the mindfire. But sometimes, emotions just need to be released. So I let myself go—and opening myself up is one of the best decisions I've ever made.

I dropped to my knees and started to hyperventilate. I collapsed down into his arms and cried, "I'm sorry I'm not the perfect girl you thought I was." All he did was hold me—quietly, peacefully, and tightly. He didn't say anything, and honestly, I didn't need him to. His silence spoke volumes. I knew he was never letting go.

I felt like a burden in showing him my baggage. He didn't deserve that. What I've learned is that we all have baggage. We're all a little broken. My boyfriend holds me and helps me breathe through panic attacks. He looks me in the eyes when I'm crying and calls me beautiful. He makes me stand in front of the mirror and tell myself everything is going to be okay. And with his arms on my shoulders, I actually believe it.

But you can't solely rely on love from your primary people. The key to combating anxiety is learning how to love yourself. I was the girl who constantly searched for love outwardly and sought validation of my worth. Heck, I wrote a whole book about guys I chased throughout my teenage years. But as I've grown into my adult self, I've started to hold my own hand. I don't love my anxiety, but I accept it. I understand that it's a part of me and always will be. My willingness to embrace my flaws with my whole heart instead of with hatred makes me a more emotionally well-rounded individual. Being able to speak openly about my anxiety and OCD has helped me establish a newfound sense of maturity.

Coping with anxiety every day can be draining. I used to have a hard time believing I could ever be happy again. But I'm finding that having anxiety only leads to living a more fulfilling life. Achievements shine brighter. Romance feels richer. Hugs are more wholesome. Since I know what it feels like to be so low, the highs are extra exciting. I wouldn't trade that for the world.

Happiness will find you. The happy days will come when you stop looking for them and just let life do its thing. Today, I graduated from college, and I felt more than just happiness. I felt hope—hope for myself and my future. The pure joy I experienced as I threw my cap in the air did more than just interrupt my anxiety. It filled me with pride. It gave me purpose. I watched my family and boyfriend waving giant cardboard cutouts of my head in the crowd. I doled out endless hugs to my best friends. I felt my late grandma's hand on my shoulder guiding me across the stage to accept my diploma. This is why we live. This is why we keep going, even when it feels impossible. We live for love. When anxiety rattles our inner peace, there will always be love.

For years, I wished my anxiety would go away. Not to sound all "doom's day," but I don't think it ever will. It doesn't get better—you just get stronger. You learn how to cope so that when anxiety does arise, you're ready to take it on. You stop running away from it and start looking it dead in the eye. To be blunt: you make anxiety your bitch. Anxiety may hurt, but it does not dictate who you are. You are more than what anxiety tells you. You are a good person. Dealing with anxiety is exhausting. It's hard. But you're still living. How lucky we are to be alive right now.

Looking back at my darkest moments, I now see that there is light. I was never a victim, and neither are you. You have the power to reframe the narrative of anxiety— let that empower you. There will be darkness. There will be rain. But the sun always rises, and light always floods back in. Make a commitment to yourself. Promise that no matter how hard it gets, you will try, and you will keep trying. You will fight for yourself, because only when you decide to never stop fighting do you when. You will keep putting one foot in front of the other, even when it feels like gravity is pulling you to the ground. You will turn pain into power that will propel you forward. You will never surrender, because there's someone out there who needs you. Life is way too beautiful not to embrace it wholeheartedly.

Day by day, breath by breath, you will persevere and prosper. Everything will be okay.

ADDITIONAL RESOURCES

Hotlines:

- If you are in crisis, reach out to the 988 Crisis Lifeline by calling or texting 988 or visiting 988lifeline.org/chat. The team provides 24/7 support and helps connect you with local mental health specialists.
- To connect with a crisis counselor, you can also text HOME to 741741.
- For additional crisis hotlines, and to find mental health professionals near you, visit https://www.apa.org/topics/crisis-hotlines.

For additional information on anxiety and OCD, or if you'd like to donate to further mental health research, please consider the organizations below.

- Anxiety and Depression Association of America: https://adaa.org
- International OCD Foundation: https://iocdf.org

- The Mental Health Coalition:
  https://www.thementalhealthcoalition.org
- National Alliance on Mental Illness:
  https://www.nami.org
- The Trevor Project:
  https://www.thetrevorproject.org
- Peace of Mind Foundation:
  https://peaceofmind.com
- Made of Millions Foundation:
  https://www.madeofmillions.com
- Not Alone Notes:
  https://www.notalonenotes.org
- NOCD:
  https://www.treatmyocd.com

ACKNOWLEDGMENTS

Although anxiety can really hurt sometimes, I'm fortunate enough to have a group of people in my life who show me unconditional love and support. This book serves as no exception.

First, I'd like to thank my parents for always being there for me—even when I try to push you away. I know I don't say it enough, but I really am so grateful for you. I may be growing up, but I promise to never turn down your hugs.

To my boyfriend, who helps me pick up the pieces when I don't have the strength to. You bring so much joy, love and light into my life. I love you.

I'd also like to thank the literary team behind *Mindfire*. Anthony, Debra, Caitlin, and Katherine, your belief in me is humbling. Thank you for letting me share my story.

I want to thank my talented book cover team: Nigel Barker, Daniela Hritcu, Janet Reynoso and Maria

Cumella. Your work is inspiring. Thank you for helping my vision come to life.

Next a special shoutout to my therapists, who will, of course, remain unnamed. You helped mold me into the person I am today. Signing up for sessions with you was one of the best decisions I've ever made.

Lastly, I'd like to thank all of you. Writing this book has not been easy, but my mission to empower each and every one of you has kept me going. I'm sending you so much love through the pages of this book. You're not alone—never forget that.

ABOUT THE AUTHOR

Carrie Berk is an NYC-based journalist, content creator, and bestselling author. Her most recent book, *My Real-Life Rom-Com*, was a Barnes & Noble bestseller and peaked at #1 in the Dating & Intimacy category on Amazon. Berk freelances for several publications, including *New York Post*, *Page Six*, *HuffPost*, *Women's Health*, and *Newsweek*.

Berk is a bestselling children's book author with twenty-one books to her credit. She penned her first book, *Peace, Love and Cupcakes*, in 2012. *The Cupcake Club* series went on to publish twelve books (selling over 300,000 copies worldwide), and became an award-winning Off-Broadway show and featured selection in 2017's New York Musical Festival. Her second series, *Fashion Academy*, stems from her passion for fashion. The six-book series also became an Off-Broadway production at Vital Theatre and is currently licensed worldwide by Concord Music Publishing. She also published a three-book series, *Ask Emma*.

She is a verified content creator with 3.8 million followers on TikTok and 880,000 on Instagram, with a combined engagement of more than 100 million. You can follow her @carrieberkk.